Fundamentals of Occupational Therapy

An Introduction to the Profession

T0386588

Fundamentals
of Occupational
Therapy

An Introduction to the Profession

Bernadette Hattjar, DrOT, MEd,
OTR/L, CWCE

Gannon University
Erie, Pennsylvania

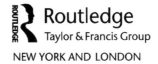

Routledge
Taylor & Francis Group

NEW YORK AND LONDON

First published in 2019 by SLACK Incorporated

Published in 2024 by Routledge
605 Third Avenue, New York, NY 10158

and by Routledge
4 Park Square, Milton Park, Abingdon, Oxon, OX14 4RN

Routledge is an imprint of the Taylor & Francis Group, an informa business

© 2019 Taylor & Francis Group

Cover Artist: Lori Shields

Library of Congress Cataloging-in-Publication Data

Names: Hattjar, Bernadette, author.

Title: Fundamentals of occupational therapy : an introduction to the profession / Bernadette Hattjar.

Description: Thorofare : Slack Incorporated, [2019] | Includes bibliographical references and index. Identifiers: LCCN 2018034746 (print) | ISBN 9781617115981 (pbk.)

Subjects: | MESH: Occupational Therapy | Occupational Therapists | United States

Classification: | LCC RM735.3 (print) | NLM WB 555 | DDC 615.8/515--dc23

LC record available at https://lccn.loc.gov/2018034746

ISBN: 9781617115981 (pbk)
ISBN: 9781003524267 (ebk)

DOI: 10.4324/9781003524267

DEDICATION

This textbook is dedicated to my family, friends, work friends, and students—both current and past. My strong support system provided me with the courage to continue working on this book and the proof that hard work really does pay off. Never give up!

CONTENTS

.

ACKNOWLEDGMENTS

This book would never have been completed without the ongoing support and understanding of everyone at SLACK Incorporated, especially Brien Cummings.

I gratefully thank my family and friends for their encouragement and prompting me to "keep going" on this book despite many personal and some professional setbacks. I am grateful to work in a supportive environment at Gannon University in Erie, Pennsylvania, and I completed this book to set a good example of diligence and focus for myself and my students.

I would certainly be remiss if I did not thank those who have passed on in my family because, at times, their divine intervention kept me going.

ABOUT THE AUTHOR

Bernadette Hattjar, DrOT, MEd, OTR/L, CWCE has been an occupational therapist since 1985. Since that time, she has worked in both the clinical and academic settings. Her experience and dedication to the field of occupational therapy moved her to consider what new, fledgling students really needed to know and understand about their field of study. The impetus for writing this textbook was an exercise in taking away, rather than adding information about the profession.

Dr. Hattjar has written and presented to professionals extensively for more than 30 years about a variety of topics including service learning, learning styles, sexuality, legacy-building opportunities, mental health issues, industrial rehabilitation practice, and intervention techniques used for pediatric clients with mental health and behavioral issues.

She has been actively involved in professional associations at the local, state, and national levels and has held the office of responsibility and leadership in these organizations.

For the past 15 years, she has taught master- and doctoral-level students in occupational therapy programs housed at Gannon University in Erie, Pennsylvania.

PREFACE

This book is the result of two divergent paths I have traveled in my personal and professional lives.

Personally, and using my more than 20 years of teaching in higher education and almost 40 years in the occupational therapy profession overall, I have never felt that such a diverse and creative field had an introductory textbook that presented a solid foundation to the profession. The textbooks that were available did not provide fledgling students with a good skill set for what was to come their way, either academically or personally. I never felt that the textbooks offered a picture of what new, incoming students needed to know. I reviewed myriad texts for the introductory course; some were quite abbreviated, and others were large and far too extensive and conceptually involved for new students. I reflected back to when I began my academic career as a new student in occupational therapy and wondered, "What did I really need to know at the onset?"

Professionally (although I realize the vastness of the profession), I have always felt that perhaps we were providing confounding information that new students would not comprehend because of their lack of a knowledge base. I also realized that students frequently confabulate information, but that doesn't necessarily mean it is correct or useful. It is just more information. If knowledge is not based on a good, solid skill set, it really isn't usable or the type of practical knowledge that one procures within the profession.

In preparing to develop and then write this textbook, I reviewed many introductory textbooks and tried to secure a clear picture of what others included, both currently and over the past 45 years. I felt that "editing" the information from current and past scholars would be an easy task. I couldn't have been more wrong. It is much easier to add than to take away pieces of information. I would constantly question and weigh out how important an item was and, in some cases, why some things were included and others were not. This was to be the bane of my existence for many months! I finally got to a point where I decided that the basics of the profession could be included in this book, but all of the minutia included in some other textbooks did not add to a welcoming introductory textbook nor was it necessary. Such specific and particular information will be presented in the curriculum classes that follow. However, students using this textbook will have a good general idea of what to expect from their occupational therapy education.

As I wrote this textbook, life happened to me, as it always does to each one of us, and each life experience taught me something about what is important and what is not. This sense provided me with a firm belief that this textbook will guide—and I hope motivate and inspire—new, incoming occupational therapy students to move forward in their academic lives.

Welcome to one of the most diverse, creative, and fulfilling professions: occupational therapy.

—*Bernadette Hattjar, DrOT, MEd, OTR/L, CWCE*

INTRODUCTION

A foundation provides stability, strength, and a point from which everything that follows is based. A building must have a solid foundation to sustain weight, stress, wear and tear, unforeseen disasters, and the effects of time. A relationship must have a solid and broad foundation to withstand whatever life presents to the individuals involved—be it positive or negative, good or bad. A profession must have a solid foundation to determine where it came from (origin and inception), where it has been (history), and where it is going (practice trends and tendencies, development, evolution). Only by understanding what comprises the foundation of any element or concept can we understand its past, present, and future.

The occupational therapy profession has a rich and diverse past that can be traced to the late 19th century. From its origin to the present, paradigms have shifted, the world has become replete with technology, and societal structure and world awareness have become blurred from the more proper and rigid concepts of the late 1800s and early 1900s to the global community of today. Interestingly, many of the original concepts on which the profession was based still hold true today, more than 100 years later. This provides evidence that the concepts and beliefs of the originators of occupational therapy were and are accurate, appropriate, and correct.

Among these tried-and-true concepts are the following:

1. Analysis of activity: Our forerunners believed that for any task to be therapeutic and both helpful and useful to the client, it had to be assessed and reduced to its smallest component parts. In our activity analysis of today, we assess a task or activity to determine its overall composition—the physical, psychological, and related components that are part of the activity—and then match the activity to our *Occupational Therapy Practice Framework* (OTPF; American Occupational Therapy Association [AOTA], 2010) to determine elements of the profession that are addressed by the activity and that apply to the client's diagnosis, needs, skills, and deficits.

2. Therapeutic use of self: Early therapists acknowledged the need to be compassionate, confidential, empathetic, informed, and attentive to the needs of the client. Today's therapists adhere to an ethical code of conduct (AOTA, 2008) and practice standards to ensure the duality of being both a professional and a service provider to individuals who are in need of our services.

3. Educational preparedness: At the dawn of the profession, the educational process was quite different from the extensive process of today's accredited occupational therapy programs (Accreditation Commission for Occupational Therapy Education, 2013); however, specific elements of physiology, anatomy, and psychology that were applicable to practice in the early 20th century still apply today. Additional educational layers of human development, human pathology, neurology, kinesiology, and abnormal psychology are included then and now to enrich and broaden the scope of knowledge. For the student, this may generally help you understand why you are taking courses within your educational program, both currently and in the future. Remember that the

scope of this profession is broad, so your knowledge and educational preparation must reflect this fact.

4. Theoretical framework: Early practice was related to a physical medicine knowledge base, a psychoanalytic and "asylum" approach to mental illness, and developmental or genetic childhood manifestations. The occupational therapy profession aligned itself with the status quo of the day, as did other health care professions. In the middle of the 20th century, occupational therapy began to develop its own theories for interventions, and this continues today. A theoretical framework provides our profession with a structured set of guidelines for evaluation, intervention, and techniques. The particular theory that is used by the therapist is reflective of the facility, the client diagnosis groups, and the vision of the organization.

5. Acknowledgment of professional differences: Occupational therapy has never thought of itself as the "be all" of health care professions or presented itself in that manner. Occupational therapy has and does work with a variety of health care providers to meet the needs of the client in a holistic, functional, and purposeful manner. It is crucial that the occupational therapy professional understand the parameters and domain of the profession. This is probably best understood by viewing the OTPF.

6. Belief in a life balance: Therapists subscribe to the belief that there must be a balance among work, rest, and leisure and play. When any of the basic elements are done to excess or not at all, the individual's life becomes "out of sync," and problems arise. In other words, too much of one thing upsets the balance in a person's life. When one adds on any illness, injury, or disability to this situation, the concept of balance and equilibrium becomes more easily understood. Both early therapists and therapists of today use a variety of intervention tools to assess and remedy a client's out-of-sync life, including a very basic checklist format of activities done during a typical day or week called an "Activity Configuration". Early practitioners believed that the mandate for structure and daily time and activity balance promoted health. This still holds true today in our busy society and in our profession.

7. Structure and consistency: Early days of the profession can be linked to 18th century Europe and "moral treatment" concepts of structure, nutrition, social and interpersonal interaction, gainful involvement in activity or tasks and chores, adequate rest, self-care and hygiene, and the development of personal levels of worth and esteem within a hospital or asylum setting. All of these things revolved around a structured, consistent schedule. Realizing that many clients had no concept of consistency and structure, the hospital or asylum structure promoted client awareness of responsibility, contributions, interaction, and self-satisfaction. This element holds true in the occupational therapy profession of the 21st century. One only needs to view a daily schedule of a client in rehabilitation to understand that the components of structure and consistency remain basic elements of client care today.

The components of the profession's past that hold true today are discussed throughout this textbook. To provide consistency and structure, each chapter is organized in the same manner. Key words are introduced at the beginning of each chapter and fully discussed and demonstrated in the specific chapter. The introduction to each chapter provides a basic history and review of specific details related to the chapter topic. History related to the chapter topic is presented for the student to understand how the specific topic or practice area has developed. "Questions to Consider for Student Learning and Reasoning" discuss appropriate evaluations and interventions that are commonly used in regard to the chapter topic. Each chapter is consolidated into the "Summary" section of each chapter as a means of both reviewing and highlighting important components for the student.

The intent of this introductory and foundational textbook is to provide entry-level occupational therapy students with the information and tools they will need to better understand, synthesize, and integrate the diverse elements of the profession into their professional-level courses, where in-depth understanding of these basic concepts occurs in an occupational therapy education program.

REFERENCES

Accreditation Commission for Occupational Therapy Education. (2013). *ACOTE standards for OTA, OTR Master and OTR doctorate programs.* Bethesda, MD: AOTA Press.

American Occupational Therapy Association. (2008). *The Occupational Therapy Code of Ethics.* Bethesda, MD: AOTA Press.

American Occupational Therapy Association. (2012). Occupational Therapy Practice Framework: Domain & process. *American Journal of Occupational Therapy, 62,* 635–682.

Introduction to the Profession of Occupational Therapy

KEY WORDS

- Activity
- Activity analysis
- American Occupational Therapy Association (AOTA)
- Client-centered approach
- Medical model
- Moral treatment
- Occupation
- *Occupational Therapy Practice Framework* (OTPF)
- Quality of life (QOL)

Hattjar, B.
Fundamentals of Occupational Therapy:
An Introduction to the Profession (pp. 1-16).
© 2019 Taylor & Francis Group.

What is occupational therapy, and how do you explain the profession to others? In 2016, the *American Occupational Therapy Association* (AOTA) defined the profession in the *Occupational Therapy Practice Framework* (OTPF) as follows:

> The practice of occupational therapy means the therapeutic use of everyday activities with individuals or groups for the purpose of participation in roles and situations in home, school, workplace, community, and other settings. Occupational therapy services are provided for the purpose of promoting health and wellness and to those who have or at risk for developing an illness, injury, disease, disorder, condition, impairment, disability, activity imitation, or participation restriction. Occupational therapy addresses the physical, cognitive, psychosocial, sensory and other aspects of performance in a variety of contexts to support engagement in everyday life activities that affect health, well-being, and *quality of life* (QOL; AOTA, 2014).

It is interesting to note that the description or definition of occupational therapy has changed over the years. For example, in 1968, occupational therapy was defined as "the art and science of directing man's response to selected activity to promote and maintain health, to prevent disability, to evaluate behavior, and to treat or train patients with physical or psychosocial dysfunction" (AOTA, 1968).

DEFINITION SIMILARITIES

Although the 1968 definition of the profession is much briefer, certain threads of similarity and difference exist between the 1968 and 2004 texts. The similarities are indicative of the underlying base of the profession: to engage those we work with in meaningful tasks designed to assist in progress or at least diminish problems. The scope of the profession is broad in that therapists work with people across the life span who experience physical, psychological, developmental, and other issues or restrictions, and this is reflected in both profession descriptions as well. Health promotion and support has and does figure prominently throughout the history of the profession, as identified in both defining statements about the profession. The well-being of those we work with is also a prominent feature of occupational therapy. This may be reflected in ongoing support of efforts and in increasing the level of independence and self-reliance that a client experiences. This improvement will be positively reflected by a client's elevated or improved quality of life. QOL is usually thought to mean an improvement or an enrichment of an individual's personal life experience.

DEFINITION DIFFERENCES

The 1968 definition of the profession seems to be somewhat restricted in scope and in the essence of the profession's domain of practice, although this is consistent with the essence of allied health professions during this time in history. This early definition describes physical and psychosocial problems, whereas the 2016 definition

---

BOX 1-1

THE MEDICAL MODEL

The medical model, according to Kielhofner (2009), was developed in and for the practice of medicine, although aspects of it are used in many health disciplines, including occupational therapy. The medical model has furthered the growth of scientific knowledge of the human body concerning biomechanical constituents of the human body and the cause-and-effect relationships, as well as the nature, causes, and management of disease and trauma (Dubos, 1959, as cited in Kielhofner, 2009, p. 235). People who work within the medical model are most concerned with the amelioration and effect of illness, injury, and disability and of returning the body into a state of homeostasis, health, and wellness.

The medical model views the client as a patient who is in need of medical treatment, and the client assumes a more-or-less passive role. The patient, in a "sick role," receives medical treatment, but his or her needs are not necessarily considered. Talcott Parsons, an American sociologist, coined the term *sick role* to describe the role patients assume when the medical model is used in health care, especially to describe the more traditional approach to illness, injury, or disability (Varul, 2017). Within this role, the "patient" relinquishes independence and becomes a passive recipient of services provided by medical staff. Services rendered by medical staff are related to correcting the effects of the injury, illness, or remediating the disability.

The patient experiences somewhat of a structured journey, moving from passivity to a cooperative relationship with more-or-less equal roles of responsibility. This is based on the patient getting better due to the medical services provided.

The medical model promotes a hierarchy of responsibility and importance or significance in regard to the patient. The coordinator, in this capacity, is usually the physician, followed by nursing interventions, then ancillary health care provider interventions, including occupational therapy. This type of stratum was common in mid-20th century medicine (Varul, 2017), but still prevails today in certain health care settings. The medical model of care is best thought of as a more conservative and traditional type of medical care.

---

encompasses a much broader range of diagnosis clusters. The 1968 definition identifies "treating and training patients," while the 2016 description of the profession uses more client-empowering and self-sufficient terminology to describe the broadness and richness of the therapy experience. The 1968 definition is more traditional and conservative in nature, but this clearly reflects the entire medical profession world of the late 1960s and the adherence to the *medical model* (Box 1-1) of care and the use of "ancillary services." The health care community of the 21st century is much more dynamic, treatment team-based, and client-centered.

Although both of these professional descriptions help to gain a large snapshot, over time, of the progression of the profession, articulating "what occupational therapy is" has and continues to be a challenging task for both novice and seasoned therapists.

The late 20th and early 21st centuries are marked by a greater understanding of what occupational therapy actually is, due to the increasing number of clients who receive or have received services with positive results. Occupational therapy has been featured in the media related to treatment of traumatic brain injury, autism or pervasive developmental disorders, the concerns of returning soldiers, spinal cord injury, and upper extremity amputations, along with involvement in mental health initiatives and treatment. Media exposure and state-of-the-art marketing endeavors by the AOTA have served to "spread the good word" about the profession.

TREATMENT TEAM

Occupational therapists work on a treatment team of professionals. A treatment team works together to share updates, thoughts, and ideas on a client's progress, or lack thereof; team members report on any problems or issues that the client is experiencing, changes in treatment, patient/client care procedures, and all other factors that will affect the client's status and discharge from a facility. This may also be referred to as a *multidisciplinary treatment team*. The team, comprising a group of diverse health care providers, meets regularly, usually once each week, to discuss their mutual clients. Members of the treatment team, including occupational therapists, each bring their discipline's perspective to the meeting. This promotes a more holistic view of the client and promotes a thorough review of the client's status in relation to each health care discipline.

To ascertain what other treatment team health care professionals "think" about the role of occupational therapy, the author interviewed a number of practicing health care professionals who are typical members of the treatment team to get their thoughts and opinions concerning "what occupational therapy is" from a practice standpoint (Patient Navigator Training, 2017).

- Speech and language pathologists work with clients who experience swallowing, feeding, or communication deficits. One such therapist felt that occupational therapy supported client feeding programs by helping identify sitting positions, wheelchair adaptations, and adaptive equipment appropriate for a particular client or groups of clients. Another speech and language pathologist felt that "the sounds and words we work on are put into action in occupational therapy."

- Social workers provide equipment necessary for a client to return home and generally serve as a liaison between the client and outside agencies, and with the family or facility. One social worker stated that occupational therapy could help a client and family by performing a home evaluation before discharge in regard to the client's home environment and need for durable medical equipment. Other social workers commented on the collaboration between occupational therapy and social work as being "helpful" and "dynamic in respect to the client's needs for returning home."

- Physicians (MDs or DOs) may be primary care physicians or specialists, depending on the setting and the clients being served. One physician stated that occupational therapy provided a broad understanding of the client as a person. This enabled the physician to gain a clearer view of client ability to move to a lesser level of care or to return to the home environment, as appropriate. Other physicians reported that occupational therapy assists clients in "learning or relearning" daily occupations and "helps clients or patients to realize that they can live life again."

- Physical therapists help clients who lack mobility, have pain, or experience functional deficits. A physical therapist reported that "working with occupational therapy ensures that any client is going to be able to be as successful and independent as possible. When we work together it's awesome and the client is the one who benefits the most." Other physical therapists stated that occupational therapists are creative and original in how they consider clients' issues and in how to resolve those issues.

- Nurses include registered nurses (RNs), licensed practical nurses, and advanced practice nurses (e.g., nurse midwifes, clinical nurse specialists, nurse practitioners). The varied role of the nurse on a treatment teams relates to their specialty and level of education and training. "Occupational therapists make my patient care easier because the patients learn to help themselves do typical things that people do each day like dressing and bathing."

THE OCCUPATIONAL THERAPY NAME: LEADING OR MISLEADING?

The term *occupation* in the profession title may be misleading: We do get other people (our clients) jobs (*occupation* usually has the connotation of a job or work), but that is one small component of this broad profession. We are not the "helpers" of other health care professions (sometimes clients may state, "You help out the other therapists"); we do work in conjunction with other professions, however. We are not the "craft people," but we do utilize crafts and creative activities with appropriate clients. We are not the "gadget people," although we utilize adaptive equipment and splints to help clients become more independent and safe in certain situations.

This highlights how important it is for the occupational therapy professionals to be able to explain exactly what occupational therapy comprises to their clients in understandable terms, not the profession's jargon. Although you may be at the beginning of your occupational therapy life role, it is time to begin to develop your own explanation of what occupational therapy is, does, and contributes to a client's well-being and health. My own script in this regard includes introducing myself and asking the client how he or she would like to be addressed. Then my explanation of occupational therapy always relates to doing tasks in the kitchen, in the bathroom, and while dressing. It then moves to home and work roles, appropriate transfers, the home situation, and the work situation, and I end by asking the client what, in his or her opinion, are the most important tasks to work on. Remember that what you may think is important may not be what a client believes is important in his or her life.

Unique to the Occupational Therapy Profession

The terminology used in the OTPF (AOTA, 2016) is important to consider both when selecting and analyzing an *activity* for client use in the evaluation and intervention processes. The OTPF identifies terminology common to the profession and identifies the professional domain of practice. *Activity analysis*, another unique component of occupational therapy, will help to determine whether the client's needs and goals can be met by the functional activity or task that the therapist selects. This is, of course, based on client strengths, limitations, and motivation.

WHAT DOES AN OCCUPATIONAL THERAPIST DO? WHAT IS UNIQUE ABOUT THE FIELD?

This section provides a practical breakdown of what occupational therapists perform in an almost automatic fashion. This is supported by the therapist's ability to critically think about the task and the client. Critical thinking is defined as "the intellectually disciplined process of actively and skillfully conceptualizing, applying, analyzing, synthesizing, and/or evaluating information gathered from or generated by observation, experience, reflection, reasoning, or communication, as a guide to belief or action" (University of Louisville, 2017). The following list describes what occupational therapists do in general terms:

- Occupational therapists support client independence through client involvement in meaningful, purposeful, goal-directed, and appropriate activities (occupations) that will either maintain or improve a client's physical, mental, or developmental health status. These activities can be creative (e.g., collage, painting, craft tasks), social/interactive (e.g., assertiveness training, social dancing, holiday events, weekly cooking of a lunch or dinner), functional (e.g., dressing, transferring, driving, cooking,), or physical (e.g., exercise or directed exercise activities or activities with a strong element of movement).

- Occupational therapists consider client interests, needs, desires, and requests to make treatment meaningful and specific to the particular client. Frequently this process is initiated by a client-centered evaluation component or through the use of an *Interest Checklist*. More recently, the AOTA has strongly supported the use of the *Activity Card Sort* (Baum, Edwards, & Gray, 2008) for obtaining the same type of information. In clinical practice, the *Activity Card Sort* and the Interest Checklist can both be used to provide a solid baseline regarding client activity interest and preference.

- Occupational therapists provide evaluation and treatment intervention(s) after carefully determining what and how the activity or task will be presented to best assist the client in becoming as independent as possible via activity analysis (our ability to break down an activity into its smallest components and match this with the OTPF terminology and practice domain).

- Occupational therapists critically think and plan for each client to achieve the best outcome, and, therefore, improve the client's QOL.
- Occupational therapists use tasks that fall within the domain of practice to attain the highest level of function as possible, despite illness, injury, or disability (providing interventions that are not too difficult or too easy means the activity has "just the right fit" for a client).
- Occupational therapists use high technology (computers, electronic devices or equipment, therapeutic modalities, etc.) or low technology (adaptive equipment, manual support items, color contrast, etc.) to support and encourage independence.
- Occupational therapists identify a theoretical approach that supports identified interventions (use of occupational therapy theories and those of other discipline that are reflected in our practice).
- Occupational therapists use both scientific and creative knowledge to support client involvement, engagement, and satisfaction in life tasks and therapeutic activities.

Many of these precepts have been a part of the profession since its inception more than 100 years ago. The reason that things have stayed the same in overall concept is because they hold true and have always provided a specific spirit to the profession that no other profession has attained. How did all of this come about? We will discuss this in the next section.

HISTORICAL EVENTS THAT SUPPORTED DEVELOPMENT OF OCCUPATIONAL THERAPY

It is helpful to understand how actual history influenced the development of the profession in the United States. The history of the profession is mirrored by the history of the United States and the development of the industrialized society. In many ways, occupational therapy was an offshoot of or a reaction to the industrialization of the United States. However, this was prefaced by factors that date back to ancient Greece and, more recently, to sentiments identified in 18th-century Europe. Industrialization, the process through which the United States moved from an agrarian society (agriculture and farming) to a society in which production and products were important, occurred during the later half of the 19th century, especially after the reconstruction of the United States after the Civil War (1861-1865). This is usually referred to as the *Industrial Revolution*. To understand how the profession was developed and grew in the United States, some historical events must be considered:

- The onslaught of immigration from Europe, Africa, and Asia during the later part of the 19th and early 20th century
- The need for the United States to produce "things" and food for its increasingly growing population

- The need for the government to export products to other countries and the need to decrease importing products from other countries, thereby increasing the financial stability and involvement in the "whole world" market and economy
- Acclamation and assimilation of different cultures into the culture of the United States. (This action forced the United States to develop its own culture. The United States became a "melting pot" of different cultures and realized the need to accommodate differences brought on by immigration.)
- The provision of some type of health care and medical intervention to the increasing population as a whole, along with the attempt to prevent communicable diseases
- The belief that people who needed health care or medical interventions should have humane and appropriate treatment, whether those problems originate in the body or the mind. (This particular precept is reflective of William Tuke's and Phillip Pinels's *moral treatment*. Moral treatment represented a new direction in health care in relation to care of those with mental illnesses in both England [Tuke] and France [Pinel]. This humanistic approach provided good nutrition, safety, structure, and a caring team of support, as opposed to somatic therapies of the day like bloodletting and of incarceration [Segen's Medical Dictionary, 2012].)
- The First World War in Europe

All of these events, occurring between the 1880s and the early decades of the 20th century, served to provide a window of opportunity for the development of the occupational therapy profession.

DEVELOPMENT OF THE PROFESSION OF OCCUPATIONAL THERAPY IN THE UNITED STATES

In the last decade of the 19th century and the first decade of the 20th century, Herbert Hall, a physician who was a strong believer in the "work cure," introduced the use of creative activity and work-related tasks into the treatment of hospitalized individuals. The effects of this "doing" process improved the physical and psychological status of these people. His ideas were based on moral treatment directives from Europe.

During the first decade of the 20th century, Susan Tracy, an RN, fostered the use of activity and trained other nurses to engage clients in what was termed *invalid occupation*. These bedside tasks, presented to invalid or bedridden clients, promoted structured and meaningful time use and a physical or psychological improvement (or both) in the status and outlook of the clients who were the service recipients. Tracy wrote a textbook for nurses, *Studies in Invalid Occupation*, in 1912. This book was what might be considered the first occupational therapy textbook, although nurses were its audience at that time. It was used to train nurses in appropriate activities that could be done at bedside, including drawing, tile crafts, small weaving projects, basketry, and the use of card and small games, among many other "bedside" or "tabletop" activities.

In 1908, Eleanor Clark Slagle, usually considered to be the "mother of occupational therapy," began her "occupational therapy" training (at age 40 years) at the Chicago School of Civics and Philanthropy in curative activities and operations. In approximately 1912, Slagle took her education to Johns Hopkins Hospital in Baltimore, Maryland, where she was appointed director of the psychiatric clinic's occupational therapy program. In this capacity, Slagle developed habit training, which was identified by the use of structure, scheduling, and meaningful tasks or occupations, and the provision of adequate food and rest, for psychiatric clients. These tasks were consistently and regularly presented, thereby becoming "habits." With the second decade of the 20th century, Slagle became more intensely involved in the founding and creation of the new occupational therapy profession.

During this same time period, William Rush Dunton, usually considered the "father of occupational therapy," introduced and implemented the use of crafts and tasks into the psychiatric program at Sheppard Asylum. In a workshop setting, clients worked on various creative and work-related tasks. Components of structure and schedules promoted control and time accountability within a psychiatric setting. In 1915, he published the book *Occupational Therapy: A Manual for Nurses*. This book provided instruction in the use of simple, portable tasks that could be used in psychiatric client treatment and further explained why the use of "activity" or "occupation" were appropriate.

George Edward Barton, an architect who experienced numerous physical and psychological challenges, was so impressed and well-rehabilitated by the use of meaningful occupation in his own hospital experience that he opened the Consolidation House, where the use of meaningful and purposeful tasks and occupations were considered to be of primary importance in client treatment, rehabilitation, and care. Barton is generally considered to be the person who first coined the term *occupational therapy*. Barton used this terminology after seeing therapists use work-related tasks or "occupations." He observed the substantial level of improvement in the clients' status, or work, and the term was applied from that point on (Watson & Wilson, 2003). Barton, as both a recipient of services and a program developer and administrator, was aware of the work of other "founding members" and made contact with Slagle, Dunton, Tracey, and Cox-Johnson (Sabonis-Chafee & Hussey, 1998).

Susan Cox-Johnson was educated as an occupational therapist, although she worked as a creative arts teacher before receiving her occupational therapy education. She infused the precepts of the early occupational therapy profession with her own educational training to formulate tasks for clients that were both creative and meaningful. Her work was so engaging and well respected that she became one of the founders of the profession.

In 1915, Canadian Thomas Kidner was appointed vocational secretary of the Canadian Military Hospital Commission. He created a system of rehabilitation programs for veterans. In his programs, the use of tasks and activities, determined to be essential and meaningful for veterans, were used. Kidner was impressed by the use of meaningful occupations in rehabilitation and created occupational therapy clinics

---

Box 1-2

FOUNDERS OF THE PROFESSION: A QUICK GLIMPSE

Eleanor Clark Slagle: Occupational therapist who received training in Chicago; moved to Baltimore to head the occupational therapy program at Shepard Asylum; one of the major therapists who promoted and developed the fledgling profession in the United States; commemorated annually, via the AOTA's Eleanor Clark Slagle Award at the association's annual conference

Susan Tracy: Registered nurse who found benefit in "invalid" or bedside activities for her clients; wrote *Studies in Invalid Occupation* in 1912 for nurse training

Susan Cox-Johnson: Art educator who became an occupational therapist; credited for her great ability to infuse both creativity and meaning in clinic tasks for her clients

Thomas Kidner: A Canadian who used occupational therapy in a vocational program for Canadian soldiers in Canadian veterans facilities

George Barton: An architect who experienced physical challenges and was so impressed with his own experiences in occupational therapy that he created the Consolidation House for rehabilitation and work-related tasks; credited with being the connection between other founders

Herbert Hall: A physician who believed in the "work cure" and instituted work-related tasks in clinics

---

within his vocational rehabilitation programs. Word of his infusion of occupational therapy into rehabilitation reached the United States and to the potential founders of the profession, and this was met with positive regard and the feeling that Kidner could be a valuable resource in the development and promotion of the profession in the United States.

In March 1917, the "founding" members of the profession met at Barton's Consolidation House, and the National Society for the Promotion of Occupational Therapy was created. In attendance at this meeting were Slagle, Dunton, Barton, Kidner, Cox-Johnson, and Isabel G. Newton, the secretary for the meeting. This was followed in September 1917 by the first general meeting of the National Society for the Promotion of Occupational Therapy (AOTA, 2017). In 1921, the name of the organization was changed to the American Occupational Therapy Association.

Although not considered to be a founding member, Adolph Meyer, a physician who historically promoted the moral and structured treatment approaches used by occupational therapists, was the keynote speaker at the first annual meeting of the AOTA.

What began as a desire to promote a kinder and more compassionate way to work with and treat people with physical or psychiatric illnesses evolved into the profession of occupational therapy (Box 1-2).

GENERAL DEVELOPMENT OF OCCUPATIONAL THERAPY: A WORLD AND HISTORICAL VIEW

Occupational therapy is based on the moral treatment of the 18th century. Moral treatment was a series of concepts and beliefs held to by Dr. Philip Pinel in France. Pinel was appalled at the inhumane treatment provided to mentally ill patients in asylums. Through his efforts and support, shackling, beating, isolation, and starvation were replaced with "moral" activities, including adequate diet and nutrition, exercise, adequate rest, involvement in purposeful tasks and activities that supported more typical life events (e.g., gardening, cleaning, self-care and grooming activities, socialization and conversation with others), and instilling a sense of safety and security (caring and compassion) for the people who resided at the asylums. This approach to care for the mentally challenged was unheard of at the time, but the results were remarkable. Patients were much easier to work with, aggressive and angry behaviors decreased, and the individuals acted more "like humans" because they were treated in a humane manner. Word of this treatment spread to England, where similar therapy was instituted by Dr. William Tuke (Quiroga, 1995). Subsequently, moral treatment reached the United States, and its concepts were instituted in Philadelphia, Boston, New York, Baltimore, and Chicago hospitals and asylums, with similar results (Quiroga, 1995). More specifically, Dr. Benjamin Rush, one of the signers of the Declaration of Independence, instituted "labor, exercise, and amusements" into the regimen of Philadelphia's Pennsylvania Hospital. Moral treatment experienced a resurgence of acceptance in the late 19th century, and in 1895, psychiatrist Dr. William Rush Dunton (nephew of Benjamin Rush) introduced activities such as metalworking and arts and crafts at Baltimore's Sheppard and Enoch Pratt Asylum.

Dr. Gary Kielhofner, in a 1992 interview for *OT Practice* magazine, stated that the precepts of moral treatment can be considered the precursor of occupational therapy (Buck, 1992), as evidenced by the implementation of these concepts into treatment by the predecessors of the occupational therapy profession in the United States. History proves this to be true.

World War I saw the development of reconstruction aides, women who were trained in occupational therapy techniques. Due to clients' excellent response to therapy activities, this was generalized to include work with injured soldiers in Europe. The reconstruction aides were sent to war zones in France, where they performed therapeutic interventions to injured soldiers. After the war, because of the high success rate and level of respect the reconstruction aides received from military personnel, occupational therapists were employed in postwar veterans and nonmilitary hospitals. Similar results from occupational therapy (now considered a viable profession) were attained during World War II. In the late 1940s, there began a force to develop a more scientific perspective (Kielhofner, as interviewed by Joe Buck, 1992), along with a move to provide more medically based interventions to a wider variety of clients, including children, the elderly, and adolescents. The 1950s saw a significant level of growth in the profession, based on both population growth and client needs in this wider and more diverse client population. The 1950s was also the decade when polio was obliterated due to Jonas Salk's vaccine, and when the first psychotropic medication, Thorazine (chlorpromazine), was developed and used to control serious mental symptoms.

To address the need for more occupational therapists, and with the acknowledgment of the particular set of skills that were needed to be a therapist (then a 4-year bachelor's degree program), the AOTA supported the development of a new technical level of practice, the certified occupational therapy assistant (COTA). COTAs received education in vocational schools or junior colleges (2-year programs). This new level of the professional culture enabled occupational therapy to expand and develop in a variety of clinical settings.

The 1960s was a time of societal change, with the glimmer of equal rights for women and the enactment of the Civil Rights and Medicare acts. The need to promote as normal a life as possible for people with psychiatric or developmental problems heralded the closing of many large state-run facilities. "Deinstitutionalization" was viewed as a positive move, and many institutionalized people were discharged from large facilities. Institutional discharge was supposed to be dovetailed with more community-based facilities to ensure consistency of care. This unfortunately did not occur in a timely manner. Many people found themselves to be ill equipped to deal with the noninstitutional world and became homeless and lacking the personal and financial resources to live in society. The burden of this situation was met by federal financial and medical assistance, the development of government-subsidized housing and apartment dwellings to meet the housing needs, and the beginning of the development of community-based health care facilities.

The 1970s saw the continuation of the societal changes that started in the 1960s. The decade also saw the beginning of health maintenance organizations (HMOs) designed to facilitate health care within a specific network of health care providers. HMOs promoted a less costly but more limited way of receiving health care to deal with the overburdened traditional health care system that was common in the United States. The 1970s also saw an increase in federal medical assistance for the growing number of underinsured or noninsured Americans. The occupational therapy profession began to experience inconsistent reimbursement for some services, based on new health insurance offerings, and developed a stronger voice in legislative endeavors.

The 1980s were a time of theoretical quandary for the profession. Traditionally, occupational therapy aligned itself as a profession, with the traditional medical model of care. The medical model of care views those we work with as "patients," and the major focus was to obliterate the illness, injury, or disability. Occupational therapists were beginning to consider the needs of their clients, but this sensibility did not have a good fit with the typical manner of health care service provision at that time in the United States. At about the same time, Canadian occupational therapists initiated a strong drive toward client-centered care, as exemplified by a change in their practice framework and through the development of the Canadian Occupational Performance Measure (a truly client-centered evaluation) and the Canadian Model of Practice. The *client-centered approach* is based in humanistic philosophy, as purported by Carl Rogers. According to Rogers, client-centeredness means that the client is the only true expert on his or her particular and personal situation (Cole, 2012). As this information filtered into the United States, therapists began to reflect on their practice model and consider the importance of a client-centered approach to practice based on the wishes, desires, and welfare of their clients. Along with this trend, there was a strong urgency to begin to control the cost of health care and provide a logical system and structure for common diagnoses. In 1986, the Diagnosis-Related Groups (DRGs) system appeared, which classifies a patient's hospital stay into various groups to facilitate payment of services. For example, the length of stay in a facility for the treatment of a particular illness, injury, or disease was determined by the national average length of patient stay for a particular illness, surgery, or disability. The health care providers needed to intervene within a certain time frame to receive insurance reimbursement. If the time frame was extended, there was no additional reimbursement for in-hospital care. Because of this issue, clients were discharged "sicker and quicker" from traditional hospitals into skilled nursing facilities, nursing homes, or home health care. For occupational therapy, this situation tended to promote a more reductionistic view of what could be accomplished due to time constraints. Conversely, the number of therapists who began to work in nonhospital settings expanded to meet the needs of the clients discharged from hospitals.

The 1990s saw a continuation of a more stringent application of DRGs. Along with this, legislation was passed to make the environment and society more accommodating to people with disabilities (the Americans With Disabilities Act, or ADA) and to increase access to services for children (Individuals with Disabilities Education Act, or IDEA). However, the large group of older Medicare recipients who received therapy services (occupational, physical, and speech therapy) experienced a significant escalation of service costs. In 1998, a capitation of therapy service charges occurred. At this time, the maximum that could be billed to Medicare per year by occupational therapy was $1,500. (However, the maximum that could be billed by physical and speech therapy was a total of $1,500 for both services). The late 1990s was the first time that therapists were losing their jobs due to these "capitation" changes. Occupational therapists are creative people and so began to create new employment arenas, including driving, living skills for a variety of client groups, doing more work with adolescents and children, and working in private therapy practices, among many other areas. These "emerging practice" areas of the late 1990s are now common practice areas for occupational therapists in the 21st century.

The onset of the 21st century has brought about a need to provide quality services in a short time frame. Therapists are acutely aware of "productivity" needs in their respective work facilities, while providing high-quality, individualized treatment. The number of occupational therapy educational programs is increasing, as is the need for more qualified therapists. The need for qualified therapists is expected to increase by almost 30% by 2030, as the baby boomer generation ages (Box 1-3) (U.S. Census Bureau, 2008). The current health care trends in the United States (2013) represent the acknowledgment that something is tragically wrong with our health care system and delivery model, and there are additional concerns when considering what can be expected for the future. Only time will tell.

BOX 1-3

GENERATIONAL NAMES AND BIRTH PERIODS

GI Generation: Aproximately 1901 to 1926

The Silent Generation: Approximately 1927 to 1945

The Baby Boomer Generation: Approximately 1945/46 to 1964

Generation X: Approximately 1964/65 to 1980

Generation Y: Approximately 1981 to 2000

Millennial Generation: Approximately 2000 to present

Isacosta Site, 2014

DEMOGRAPHICS

The need for occupational therapists and occupational therapy assistants is expected to remain strong through the first decades of the 21st century. The U.S. Bureau of Labor Statistics (2014) indicates that there will be an increased demand for therapists between now and 2022 of 29%; in numbers, this means that there will be an increased need for more than 32,000 occupational therapy practitioners during this time period. Job growth will be "much faster than average" (U.S. Bureau of Labor Statistics, 2014). This fast growth rate mandates an increased need for more therapy educational programs at both the professional level (registered occupational therapists) and the technical level (occupational therapy assistant). The need for additional practitioners requires an increased number of educational programs. In 2014 to 2015, the number of occupational therapy accredited education programs in the United States was as follows (AOTA, 2015):

- Doctoral level: 7
- Masters level: + 159 (183)
- Technical level: + 213 (260)

SUMMARY

Compared with many other professions, both within and outside of the health care arena, occupational therapy is still in its infancy. During the past 100 years, the profession has developed, expanded, changed, and attempted to meet the needs of an ever-changing population demand. This has been expressed by the changing scope of practice, education, and the development of professional theories and techniques. Through this century of occupational therapy, and although many things have changed, we as a profession still hold firm to the original concepts and beliefs of our creators. Because of this strong and solid professional base, the profession has become firmly entrenched in the health care arena in the United States and will continue to be a preeminent component of holistic health care in the future.

QUESTIONS TO CONSIDER
FOR STUDENT LEARNING AND REASONING

1. In what ways does the diversity of the founding members of the profession help to define occupational therapy?
2. How did the overall scope of the young profession define what we do in occupational therapy today, more than 100 years later?
3. Identify some areas that occupational therapy can discuss in treatment team meetings for clients that other disciplines cannot.
4. In relation to other disciplines, identify other health care professions that help support occupational therapy in providing holistic and thorough care for a client.

REFERENCES

American Occupational Therapy Association. (2017). *Important events from 1960-1969.* Retrieved from: http://www.otcentennial.org/events/1960

American Occupational Therapy Association. (2017). *Important events from 1917.* Retrieved from: http://www.otcentennial.org/events/1910

American Occupational Therapy Association. (2015). *Academic programs annual data report 2014-2015.* Retrieved from: https://www.aota.org/~/media/Corporate/Files/EducationCareers/Educators/2014-2015-Annual-Data-Report.pdf

American Occupational Therapy Association. (2014). *Occupational therapy practice framework: Domain & process* (3rd ed.). Bethesda, MD: AOTA Press.

Baum, C., Edwards, D., & Gray, M. (2008). *Activity Card Sort* (2nd ed.). Bethesda, MD: AOTA Press.

Buck, J. (1992, March 28). Humane treatment: A foundation for the profession. *OT Week,* pp. 14-15.

Chillemi, T. (2018). An Introduction to the Healthcare System. Retrieved from: http://patientnavigatortraining.org/introduction-to-the-healthcare-system/

Cole, M. (2012). *Group dynamics in occupational therapy.* Thorofare, NJ: SLACK Incorporated.

Dubos, R. (1959). *The mirage of health.* New York, NY: Harper & Row.

Dunton, W.R. (1915). *Occupation Therapy: A Manual for Nurses.* Philadelphia, PA: W.B. Saunders.

Isacosta Site. (2014). *List of generations chart.* Retrieved from: http://wwwesds.l.pt

Kielhofner, G. (2009). The medical model. In G. Kielhofner (Ed.), *Conceptual foundations of occupational therapy practice* (4th ed.). Philadelphia, PA: F.A. Davis.

Matsutsuyu, J.S. (1969). The interest checklist. *American Journal of Occupational Therapy,* 23, 323-328.

Novak, J. (2018). *The Six Living Generations in America.* Retrieved from: http://www.marketingteacher.com/the-six-living-generations-in-america/?highlight=six%20living%20generations

Quiroga, V. (1995). *Occupational therapy: The first 30 years.* Bethesda, MD: AOTA Press.

Patient Navigator Training. (2017). Retrieved from http://www.patientnavigatortraining.org/healthcare_system/module

Sabonis-Chaffee, B., & Hussey, S. (1998). *Introduction to occupational therapy* (2nd ed.). St. Louis, MO: Mosby-Year Book.

Segen's Medical Dictionary. (2012). *Moral treatment.* Farlex, Inc. Retrieved from https://medical-dictionary.thefreedictionary.com/moral+treatment

Tracy, S.A. (1912). *Studies in Invalid Occupation: A Manual for Nurses and Attendants.* Boston, MA. Whitcomb & Banas.

University of Louisville. (2017). *What is critical thinking?* Retrieved from http://louisville.edu/ideastoaction/about/criticalthinking/what

U.S. Bureau of Labor Statistics. (2014). *Occupational outlook handbook, 2014–2015.* Retrieved from http://www.bis.gov/ooh/healthcare/occupational_therapists.htm

U.S. Census Bureau, (2008). *Baby boomer population.* Retrieved http://www. uscensusbureau.org

U.S. Department of Labor Statistics. (2014). Occupational Therapy Outlook Handbook. Retrieved from: http://www.usdeptoflaborstatistics.org

Varul, M. (2017). Talcott Parsons, the sick role, and chronic illness. *Body & Society, 16,* 72-94.

Watson, D., & Wilson, S. (2003). *Task analysis: An individual and population approach.* Bethesda, MD: AOTA Press.

Practice in Mental Health and Psychosocial Occupational Therapy

KEY WORDS

- Deinstitutionalization
- *Diagnostic and Statistical Manual of Mental Disorders* (DSM)
- Mind-body connection
- Projective techniques
- Psychotropic medications
- Sick role
- Stigma

Hattjar, B.
*Fundamentals of Occupational Therapy:
An Introduction to the Profession* (pp. 17-32).
© 2019 Taylor & Francis Group.

The concept of the *mind-body connection* (Renoir, Hasebe, & Grey, 2003) is an important concept for occupational therapy students to understand. Within our profession, it is best to keep this thought at the forefront of your therapy tools Remember that if the body is not functioning well, the mind follows suit; if the mind is not functioning well, the body follows suit.

Psychosocial practice in occupational therapy has been an element of the profession since its starting point 100 years ago and was once a major area of employment for occupational therapists. The profession's involvement in mental health fell drastically in the latter part of the 20th century due to a number of factors, including the use of *psychotropic medications*; decreasing, limited, or low insurance reimbursement for occupational therapy; less interest in the psychosocial or mental health aspects within the profession; and few potential clinical site placements for fieldwork rotations and employment in the area. Currently, the American Occupational Therapy Association (AOTA) has an expressed focus to bolster and renew interest and practice in the psychosocial area of the profession. With current health care directions such as community-based interventions, the greater understanding of the impact of our societal demands on the human psyche, and a reduction in the *stigma* (a negative label) associated with mental health problems, access and utilization of mental health offerings is increasing—much to the benefit of millions of people. The AOTA (2014) has stated that "mental health (issues or problems) will be the top cause of disability—specifically depression. Mental health practice will be a vital practice area for the 21st century, especially for children youth and the elderly." This coincides with the profession's *Centennial Vision* (AOTA, 2006) for the future direction and focus on mental health practice in occupational therapy.

PSYCHOSOCIAL PRACTICE

Psychosocial practice has moved from a "traditional" hospital or inpatient setting to less traditional outpatient and community-based environments. Before the mid-1960s, the majority of occupational therapy clients seeking evaluation and treatment for mental health problems secured services in general hospitals, psychiatric units, or in facilities focused solely on the treatment of mental health problems (mental hospitals). In the early 1960s, an expressed mandate to "deinstitutionalize" people with mental health problems occurred, culminating in 1963 with the enactment of the Community Mental Heath Act (AOTA, 2014). Since that time, the focus of psychosocial occupational therapy has been to provide services outside of hospital settings. Currently, therapists who are employed in this area provide work in their community at a variety of setting areas including but not limited to the following:

- Community centers
- Homeless shelters
- Women's shelters
- After school programs for children, youth, and adolescents
- Senior centers

- Consumer-operated service centers
- Client homes
- Worksites
- Correctional facilities
- Psychosocial clubhouses (AOTA, 2014), which are consumer-driven, community-based agencies

This does not mean that evaluation and interventions located in inpatient settings have been eliminated. Occupational therapists may provide evaluation and recommendations for clients admitted to an inpatient psychiatric unit, but due to clients' short length of stay (at the most 3 to 5 days for observation, evaluation, and medication management), actual intervention is difficult, if not impossible, to accomplish. In many cases, clients are transferred to a lesser level of care in community-based agencies where structured and ongoing therapy interventions can occur over a period of time.

At its inception and historically, the Community Mental Health Act of 1963 focused primarily on getting mental health clients out of the artificial world of the hospital. It was determined that the actual hospital environment thwarted and severely limited the normalization of the psychiatric clients. The drive, therefore, was to move these people back into society and the community. *Deinstitutionalization* (ie, getting clients into the community and out of the institution) outpaced the development of, and funding for, needed community sites and services, as well as adequate housing, and many of these people became homeless (Accordino, Porter, & Morse, 2001). In spirit, the original concept appeared to be a good idea. In reality, these patients had few resources to be successful in the real world. The secondary effect of this situation resulted in many occupational therapists losing their jobs. This situation resulted in other health care professions "rebounding" into policy and decision making about these deinstitutionalized clients, but this was not the case for occupational therapy (Gutman, 2011).

The patient deficits were magnified by the actual environmental and community deficits in relation not only to housing, but to support, work, time utilization, and familiarity with functioning in society not within an institution. There were insufficient community-based supports and treatment programs, resulting in a disconnect between the patient's life in a structured hospital society and the patient's life in society and the community. The presence and increasing numbers of group homes, sheltered work places, and community-based programs has partially addressed the number of community-dwelling, minimally prepared or ill-equipped clients since this time but continues to be insufficient. Therefore, the work of the occupational therapy practitioner has moved from the traditional hospital setting where the "medical model" of care and the placement or assignment of the patient into a *"sick role"* predominates, to the community where the recovery model and rehabilitation models of care are present and experiencing a slight increase in occupational therapy practice. Box 2-1 compares the medical model with the recovery and rehabilitation models, and Box 2-2 describes the "sick role."

BOX 2-1

THE MEDICAL MODEL COMPARED WITH
THE RECOVERY AND REHABILITATION MODELS

MEDICAL MODEL

The medical model of patient or client care places a hierarchical structure within more traditional and hospital-based settings. It applies to psychosocial and physical diagnosis patient groups. The main focus of the medical model is the amelioration of illness, disease, or injury. Clients are viewed as being sick and are not responsible or able to make decisions about their care. This coincides with Stephanie Medley-Rath's (2012) *sick role*. In a sick role, the physician or health care providers, not clients, are viewed as the experts on the disease, illness, or injury entities that are present. Clients permit health care professionals (doctors, surgeons, nurses, therapists, etc.) to take the lead in their treatment and assume a passive role in their own care. "Get the person well" is the focus of the medical model. However, as clients' health improves, their role increases because they are illness-free and have more of an ability to negotiate their treatment.

RECOVERY MODEL

This model of care seeks to engage and involve patients/clients in their treatment to varying degrees, depending on their individual status. The recovery model is used when a client is placed in a "different" environment and must learn to function within different levels of care or support, all done within the confines of one's illness, injury, or disease.

REHABILITATION MODEL

In psychosocial occupational therapy, the rehabilitation model seeks to help the client acquire skills and behaviors needed to exist outside an institution (Edelsen, 1996) or in the community. King (Edelsen, 1996) stated that this model seeks to help a client exist "at the individual's maximum level of independence, productivity, and happiness." This includes occupational responsibilities and roles at work and home; in the community; with finances, housekeeping, and relationships; and in all other components of an individual's life.

BOX 2-2

THE SICK ROLE

The concept of the patient's "sick role" was presented by Talcott Parsons, a social scientist, in the mid-20th century. Parsons believed that illness was a dysfunctional deviance comprising four specific norms: (1) the individual is not responsible for the illness, (2) the inability to fulfill normal obligations become excusable for the individual, (3) illness is undesirable, (4) those who are ill should seek professional help (Hughes, 1996). Within this context, the patient assumes the sick role until social reintegration (rehabilitation, habilitation, or the absence of illness or disease) is attained. The sick role may be passive, with the health care provider taking control, or it may include a shared decision-making process (Stiggelbout & Kiebert, 1997) in which the patient and provider work cooperatively. The shared decision-making process represents a departure from the traditional medical model.

To further substantiate the move toward the recovery and rehabilitation models, the AOTA conducted systematic reviews in the first decade of the 21st century (D'Amico, Jaffe, & Gibson, 2010; Gutman, 2012). These reviews indicate the paucity of research and published studies related to mental health occupational therapy. Almost 50% of the studies published in the *American Journal of Occupational Therapy* from 2008 through 2011 that dealt with mental health issues were conducted outside the United States (United Kingdom, Australia, Canada, Israel, Taiwan, & Hong Kong; Gutman, 2012). This highlights the current standing and relevance of mental health/psychosocial practice in occupational therapy. AOTA's *Centennial Vision* (2006) expresses the need to promote, and perhaps reestablish, mental health as a viable and necessary component of occupational therapy professional practice, further underlining the importance of this area of practice.

THE OCCUPATIONAL THERAPY PRACTITIONER IN THE PSYCHOSOCIAL ARENA

The work focus in psychosocial occupational therapy is varied. Because of the strong community-based focus, the variability is limited only by the number of community-based settings that are present. Obviously, there are currently many more work options available in more populated areas and fewer options in areas with low population or rural settings.

To be successful, the occupational therapist who works in the psychosocial area of practice must have a good level of understanding about the variety of diagnoses groups that may be seen, along with a strong knowledge base of the particular diagnosis. Additionally, psychosocial occupational therapists must have a varied selection of tasks and activities at hand; be comfortable and skilled in conducting client groups and individual sessions; and have a clear picture of who they are regarding their feelings, biases, and experiences. To provide community-based services, occupational therapists must also have a clear understanding of available community resources for these clients. In other words, "Therapist, know thyself!"

MAJOR DIAGNOSIS GROUPS COMMONLY SEEN IN PSYCHOSOCIAL OCCUPATIONAL THERAPY

The major diagnosis groups seen in psychosocial occupational therapy mirror the diagnosis groups identified in the fourth edition (with text revision) and fifth edition of the *Diagnostic and Statistical Manual of Mental Disorders* {DSM–IV–TR [American Psychiatric Association] (APA), 2004; DSM–5 (APA) 2013}. These diagnoses, placed in a structure called a *spectrum* (APA, 2013) in which diagnosis are viewed in relation to the severity and persistence of symptoms, rather than by a name (to

---

BOX 2-3

PERSONALITY DISORDER CLUSTERS

These personality type clusters will help you to understand the scope of these lifelong disorders. Although these individuals may move more freely within society, they tend to not respond well to any medication. Personality is a factor we are born with, and this factor remains more or less constant throughout life. In some situations, the disordered personality symptoms may increase or decrease if the individual is under stress or is experiencing a life-altering situation like a severe illness or the death or loss of a loved one. The particular names associated with the three clusters are terms frequently used in the "real" clinical world and come from the DSM-IV-TR rather than the current DSM-5. Do understand that the DSM-IV-TR was the "gold standard" for many years within the psychiatric setting.

- Cluster A: These individuals are identified with odd and/or eccentric personalities and are viewed as being isolated, preoccupied, distressed, and tend to have little if any social support; diagnosis names are schizotypal, schizoid, and paranoid.

- Cluster B: These individuals are dramatic and emotional. Consider the phrase, "it's all about me" and you will have an idea of this clusters' tendencies. Diagnoses within this cluster include antisocial, borderline, and histrionic personality types. Cluster B personality types behave in manners that reflect positively on the individual, not others usually, yet they are dependent on others and seek the approval or attention of others.

- Cluster C: These personality types tend to be anxious and fearful and may feel internally divided or, "at war" with themselves. Diagnoses associated with this cluster include avoidant, dependent, and obsessive-compulsive personalities. This cluster of individuals may seek out the support of others to diminish their anxiety and fear of being alone or of being "found out" in regard to their actions or words.

---

avoid the stigma of a label), include but are not limited to the following (APA, 2013; Bonder, 2015):

- Psychotic disorders: schizophrenia and all subtypes
- Mood disorders: major depression, mania, bipolar disorders, cyclothymia, hypo-mania, depressive episodes
- Anxiety disorders: panic attacks, panic disorders, unspecified anxiety disorders, separation anxiety
- Personality disorders: diagnoses identified in the three major clusters of personality disorders (Box 2-3)
- Disorders of infancy and childhood: autism, autism spectrum, pervasive developmental disorders, intellectual deficiencies (formerly mental retardation), motor and speech problems, learning deficiencies
- Diagnoses associated with aging: dementia, including dementia of the Alzheimer's type, delirium
- Disorders commonly seen in childhood or adolescence include: oppositional defiant disorder, conduct disorder, learning disorders, social phobias, substance abuse, suicide
- Disorders associated with adulthood: depression, anxiety, sexual dysfunction disorders

Box 2-4

THE OCCUPATIONAL THERAPY PROCESS IN PSYCHOSOCIAL OCCUPATIONAL THERAPY

1. Referral is secured from a physician or other health care professional; this process occurs on a state-by-state basis.

2. Screening is usually a brief interaction designed to assess the client's cognition, memory, interaction, and understanding of structured questions.

3. Evaluation and assessment is performed by the registered occupational therapist and guided by the client and client needs. Under the supervision of the registered occupational therapist, the certified occupational therapy assistant may be called on to perform some of the more technical components of the evaluation, for example, an activities of daily living (ADL) assessment for dressing or grooming.

4. Goals are determined based on evaluation and screen results.

5. A client treatment plan is developed that identifies the specific course of intervention and individual client needs.

6. Client interventions and therapy begin, aligned with the treatment plan or plan of care.

7. Client reevaluation includes goal updates or elimination (if a goal has been attained). This is usually conducted at least every 2 weeks or more frequently.

8. Client discontinuation or discharge with recommendations for continued care options: the discontinuation of services at one level of care is usually followed by the client securing services in a lesser care setting (for example, if a client is seen in an inpatient setting, services may be secure in an outpatient, community-based facility, in a partial hospital setting, or elsewhere)

Only two of these diagnoses are considered to be lifelong in nature or persistence: personality disorders and intellectual deficiencies. This is reinforced by both the DSM–IV–TR and the currently used DSM–5.

Referral

To provide any therapeutic evaluation or intervention, occupational therapists must secure a physician's order or referral (Box 2-4). In a traditional setting, this would include "orders" identified on the client medical chart. In a community setting, this may include receiving a prescription form from a physician or referral agency or any similar type of "hard copy" documentation requesting occupational therapy. Frequently, the orders for therapy state that the therapist must "evaluate and treat" for a specific issue or occupational deficit. The clearer the orders, the easier it becomes to determine what will occur in the evaluation process and in treatment. If the therapist has any questions about the referral or what is requested, he or she must contact the physician or referral source for clarification before proceeding to ensure quality and consistency of care.

Screening

Frequently, the occupational therapist or occupational therapy assistant may conduct a simple, brief screen to determine client orientation, as an introductory encounter, or to determine the clients' status, appearance, and other characteristics before a formal evaluation occurs. On occasion, the screen may result in the client not requiring services or being unable to tolerate services. If the client can and does require evaluation, it is scheduled. If the client cannot tolerate or does not require services, this would be documented and reported back to the referral source and other involved health care professionals. Screens that are commonly used in occupational therapy include the Mini-Mental State Examination (Mini-Mental State Examination, 1975) and the Allen Cognitive Level Screen (Allen, Austin, Earhart, McCrath, & Riska, 2007) or diagnosis-specific screens available at the Substance Abuse and Mental Health Service Administration (SAMHSA) website http://www.integration.samhsa.gov. Like the SAMHSA screen, the Mini Mental State Examination (MMSE). is in the public domain and may be accessed online.

Evaluation and Assessment

Evaluation follows the screening process. Many facilities develop their own unique evaluation for their particular clients. Other facilities use standardized assessments such as the Kohlman Evaluations Living Skills (for ADL; Kohlman, 1992), the Bay Area Functional Performance Evaluation (used to determine a variety of problem-solving and skill-based attributes; Williams & Bloomer, n.d.); an age-appropriate version of the Sensory Profile (to determine sensory processing and preference issues; Brown & Dunn, 2002; Dunn, 1999), the Lowenstein Occupational Therapy Cognitive Assessment (LOTCA), the D-LOTCA (for individuals who have experienced traumatic brain injury or have cognitive deficits; Katz, Bar-Haim, Livini, & Averback, 2013), or LOTCA-G (for older people; used to assess a variety of cognitive, organization, and skill set issues; Itzkovick, Averbuch, Elizer, & Katz, 1996, 2000); the Adolescent Role Assessment (for adolescents and adolescent-related issues; Black, 1976); or the Childhood Autism Rating Scale (for children or youth who experience autism-like features or to rule out autism in a differential diagnosis; Schropler & Bourgondien, 2010). Additionally, some facilities will use a combination of their own evaluation and a standardized evaluation; this determination is made by the facility. The evaluation should directly relate to the client age and stage, as well as the diagnosis, for it to be meaningful and appropriate.

Problem Identification and Goal Setting

Once screening and evaluation are completed, the therapist must determine the most appropriate treatment goals, which relate to the client, client needs, client's expressed interests, and client's life. Client goals should always be written in the typical "behavioral goal" formula:

- A goal must be understandable.
- A goal should be measureable.
- A goal or work on the goal should be observable.
- A goal should be objective.
- A goal should have a time frame for completion.

These guidelines apply for any occupational therapy goal, with any client group, in any setting. Goals are generally divided into long-term goals (e.g., larger content goals that will take a longer period of time to completely meet) and short-term goals (best thought of as inherent parts or components of the overall long-term goal) (Box 2-5).

At this point, the preparatory work for intervention has been accomplished.

Treatment Planning

Planning treatment for any client is challenging. Because occupational therapy purports to be a client-centered profession, client needs and interests must be considered, as occurred in the evaluation. A thorough, comprehensive, and engaging way to determine the client's personal current and previous interests, along with identification of activities and things a client would be interested in executing in the future, is the Interest Checklist. The Interest Checklist is an exhaustive form that can be completed independently or read to the client. It provides the therapist with additional information that can guide treatment interventions (Matsutsuyu, 1969. Additionally, the use of the Canadian Occupational Therapy Performance Measure (Canadian Association of Occupational Therapy, 1992) may be of value. In this client-centered assessment, clients are asked, in a conversational format, what is important to them and how satisfied they are with their performance of specifically client-identified problems or issues.

With the screen, evaluation, and identification of problems and interests completed, it is time to plan client treatment interventions based on the preparatory work that has occurred.

INTERVENTIONS

Interventions can be accomplished on either a one-on-one basis or in small groups. Some clients will not be amenable to group work initially; therefore, meeting individually can promote trust and the development of a positive and constructive therapeutic relationship with the therapist. Once the client is amenable to small group work, group topics and activities planned by the therapist can begin.

In psychosocial occupational therapy, therapists frequently adopt a group format. Group work is activity- or task-based and is defined as "a series of linked episodes of task performance by an individual which takes place on a specific occasion during a finite period for a particular reason" (Creek, 2003, as cited by Bullock & Bannigan, 2011). The activity or task topic of any group is usually determined by the needs of

---

Box 2-5

Occupational Therapy Goal Writing

Goal writing should be a concise, clear way of writing goals related to client performance. Goals are best thought of as being objective, observable, and measurable and should have a clear time frame. The following items are composites of how a behavioral goal should be written, but they exemplify the structure for how to write any goal. In the current health care arena, goals should be written in this manner to ensure the therapist of insurance company reimbursement.

Examples:

1. John will verbally share his feelings about group involvement at least once during each occupational therapy group session by December 22 (timeline for weekly note for December 16).

2. Mary will assume leadership roles in occupational therapy groups by handing out and keeping account of craft items needed for activities. She will also account for returned items and replace them in the sharps cabinet before each group is dismissed over the next 2 weeks.

3. Suzi will independently complete morning dressing, bathing, and grooming tasks and will account for her performance on her ADL Checklist daily. The occupational therapist will review her performance of these tasks each morning.

As you can see, these goals are objective (either they are completed or not completed), observable (these tasks can be viewed or questioned about for answers), measurable (to what extent were they done or not done; how many times, etc.), and include a specific time frame for completion. The more specific your goals are, the better!

Goals can also be thought of as long term and short term. Long-term goals state the overarching "big" topic to be addressed, whereas short-term goals represent tasks that comprise the long-term goal. For example, if your goal is to increase ADL performance, your short-term goals could identify parts of ADL such as dressing, bathing, hygiene, dental care, and toileting. If your long-term goal is to improve attention level, your short-term goals could address attention components such as structure, following steps in a task, increasing the amount of time the client performs a task, and being able to focus on a task without starting and stopping or requiring redirection, for example. Generally, as short-term goals are met, the long-term goal becomes more attainable for the client.

---

the particular client group. For example, a group designed to help clients who will be embarking on the job interview process will be helpful for clients seeking employment; this would be less meaningful to clients who are not seeking employment.

Occupational therapists generally believe that activity groups are more effective than "verbal" groups for developing interpersonal skills (Denton, 1997). Estelle Breines (1995), a noted occupational therapist, stated that "human beings define their lives, cultures, and worth through activities." This concept is supported by another noted occupational therapist, Marilyn Cole (2012), who talks about the dyadic relationship that occurs within a group. The dyadic process refers to the doing process involved in the group learning and doing component and also by the social and interaction component that occurs when any individual does something with another person or group of people.

Generally, intervention activities can be divided into three major areas: (1) physical and recreational, (2) creative and projective, and (3) social and interactional. Every activity falls, more or less, into one of these categories.

Physical and Recreational Activities

These are best thought of as the activities that involve gross motor, visual motor, and fine motor skills, along with components of balance, motor planning, speed and agility, endurance, intact range of motion, and the expiation of calories. The client may be experiencing diminished physical abilities, and these types of activities address physical and motor limitations. Some examples of these types of activities are competitive sports, physical games, picnic or party games, exercise, strength-building activities, and aerobic activities. These can be done in teams or individually and can be highly or minimally competitive.

For children, these types of activities might include obstacle courses, volleyball, kickball, softball, Wiffle ball or baseball, touch or tackle football, flag football, soccer, basketball, or track-and-field activities. For this group of clients, playground activities like riding a seesaw, sliding down a sliding board, or twirling on a merry-go-round can also be considered. Sometimes these activities for younger people can be those included in school gym classes, such as rope climbing, tag-team relays, and tumbling or rolling. For adolescents, the focus may be more on the refinement of physical skills and health and wellness activities, including dancing, exercise for flexibility or to improve posture, trampoline, yoga, Pilates, and exercise videos. For adults, a wide variety of activities, based on clients' interests, can be accomplished. This can include, multilayered activities such as health and wellness offerings based on weight control and reduction of caloric intake; regulation of a healthy body mass index through healthy and wise food selection and exercise; a walking, jogging, or running group; and competitive sport activities, including activities described for other age-groups, along with tennis, golf, and bicycling. For older adults, physical and recreational activities can include yoga, tai chi, stretching and range of motion activities, dancing, picnic and party games, and other less resistive tasks.

Creative and Projective Activities

This category can include a wide variety of activities that promote creativity and the expression of emotions that the client cannot readily verbalize. These activities usually comprise painting, drawing, crafting, dancing, performing or acting, writing, needlework activities, woodworking activities, leatherworking activities, cooking or baking tasks, and journaling or reminiscing. In some settings, ceramics, metalwork, and sewing are used. For these types of activities, equipment and supply costs must be considered because they can become expensive.

Projective activities, more frequently and commonly used in the 1950 through 1970s, are included through the use of life lines, the House-Tree-Person assessment, a kinetic family drawing, or magazine picture collages, used either as an activity or an assessment. For clients who cannot verbally express feelings and emotion related to disturbing occurrences in their lives, *projective techniques* can both depict and mobilize feeling for the purposes of expiation, understanding, awareness, and acknowledgment. It is important to stress to clients that they are not expected to be fine artists; it is the content of their creative productions that is important.

Social and Interactional Activities

These activities have the expressed focus of improving socialization skills and promoting improved interpersonal interaction. They can be socially focused, such as parties, dances, or cooking activities, or focused on the acquisition of skills, as in assertiveness training, public speaking, interviewing techniques (for a job, dealing with employees, or with family members), or social gathering activities such as meetings or religious events or services, to name only a few of the plethora of potential activities. These can essentially be focused on "learning" skills, relearning skills, expanding on one's current skills, or updating skills (i.e., keyboarding on a computer compared with a typewriter). Many times, social and interaction elements of activities become primary rather than secondary. This means that the interaction element(s) become more evident than the intent of the activity (e.g., playing a card game or a cooking or baking activity).

Reevaluation

Reevaluation of any client should occur on a regular basis and at least every 2 weeks. A reevaluation examines the original goals and needs, determines client progress made to date, and reports this information to the referral source and other health care professionals who work with the client. If treatment goals are met, new, updated goals can be introduced as appropriate. Once the client has met all treatment goals and is functioning in a more independent and symptom-free mode, the client's involvement in occupational therapy is discontinued.

Discontinuation or Discharge

First, "discontinuation" and "discharge" are not to be used interchangeably. Discontinuation means that the client no longer requires occupational therapy services and is discontinued from therapy. The reasons for discontinuation must be clearly stated. Discharge, in contrast, means that the client is no longer receiving any services. It is crucial to remember that these terms represent different end points for a client.

When services are discontinued, the particular needs for the clients' future care, housing disposition, support situation, and work or financial status should be laid out in an understandable manner. This information is shared with other health care professionals. It is also important to document the client's pre- and post-functional status when services are no longer determined to be necessary. This information comes from the client's goals and progress notes.

THEORIES THAT GUIDE PRACTICE

A variety of occupational therapy theories, as well as theories from other disciplines, guide practice in the psychosocial area of occupational therapy practice. These are discussed at length in Chapter 5 but are provided here in general terms:

- Client-centered theory (humanistic theory/existentialism): This approach for practice relies on the held truth that the client is the only expert on his or her situation.
- Behavioral theory (based in psychology and used if occupational therapists are focusing on clients' behavioral change): This approach includes components of reinforcement of positive or desired behaviors and the elimination or lessening of behaviors that are not positive or productive (e.g., anger, anxiety, isolation, emotional instability).
- Cognitive theory: This approach is used to assess and improve, if appropriate, a client's cognitive status or to decrease the likelihood of cognitive function decreases. It promotes improved interaction, communication, memory, and engagement in life tasks, for example.
- Developmental theory: This approach is used to promote performance and engagement closer to a client's appropriate age and stage. It helps determine the effects of illness, injury, or disability on developmental progression and engagement in developmentally appropriate tasks and activities.
- Model of Human Occupation (MOHO): This approach is used to enable clients to experience how they interpret, respond to, and act of environmental information. It assists clients in improving their ability to function and participate in living skills. The MOHO feedback loop consists of (a) input from the external environment; (b) throughput—how this external information is processed internally in regard to habits, personal perspectives and how we see and experience things, and our level of receptivity; and (c) how our internal processes influence our output to the environment (our response). This process influences the feedback we receive as input and continues over and over again. The MOHO is a dynamic approach because each person has a dynamic experience in his or her life that proceeds in an ongoing basis. The MOHO is more general in content and can be used with other theoretical bases or alone and can also be used, more or less, throughout the life span, although it is best used with older adolescents or adults because of the maturity and life experiences encountered by individuals in these age-groups.
- Intentional relationship approach: This enables therapists to gain a clear perspective on how and what they contribute to the therapist-client therapeutic relationship. The theory suggests that the therapeutic relationship between a client and a therapist sets the stage for the promotion of health, wellness, and both interpersonal and environmental interaction. This approach can be likened to the now-outmoded terminology *therapeutic use of self*. The terminology understood by many occupational therapists as the "therapeutic use of self" but is now frequently referred to as the therapeutic, intentional relationship or intentional

relationship. The intentional relationship approach places great value on the therapist knowing the self, understanding the perspective of the client or patient, respect and consideration for the client or patient, ethical treatment of the client or patient, and the confidentiality and empathy aspects of this relationship.

CASE STUDY FOR PSYCHOSOCIAL OCCUPATIONAL THERAPY

John, a 63-year-old divorced man, resides alone in a townhome. He had to stop working recently due to a recurrent bout with depression, along with the effects of degenerative joint disease, commonly seen with the aging process. John is aware of his symptoms: sleeplessness, lack of energy, anhedonia (inability to feel pleasure for tasks, interaction with people, the environment), weight gain, and preoccupation with "everything I have ever done wrong in my life." He does not take his antidepressant medication on a consistent basis and prefers to be alone in his townhome. He watches television, listens to what he describes as "sad" music, and eats "a lot of junk food." John was referred to occupational therapy by his psychiatrist for medication management, evaluation, and "suggestions for referral to a community-based treatment program" and for assessment of his self-care skills and household management skills and safety level.

1. On the basis of the occupational therapy process, identify the initial step in your work with John.
2. Identify one or two assessments or evaluations identified in this chapter that would look more closely at the problems John is experiencing.
3. Because John isolates himself from others, what would be an appropriate tool that could be used to identify interests and promote a more active use of leisure time?
4. If John used to like to play cards, cook, and walk around his neighborhood, what tasks could you provide in interventions?
5. What kind of community-based facility might be a beneficial referral for this client?

SUMMARY

The occupational therapy profession has its roots in the psychosocial health care arena. Even in the early days of the profession, the aspect of doing and engaging clients/patients in health-producing tasks or activities was noted to bring about positive changes within the population. Throughout the 20th century, involvement in the psychosocial aspect of occupational therapy lessened due to the use of psychotropic medication, legislation, and the reduction in payment for services. In recent years, a more positive focus on the resurgence of psychosocial occupational therapy has become evident with the AOTA *Centennial Vision* and the increasing need to address cultural and societal mental health issues.

QUESTIONS TO CONSIDER FOR STUDENT LEARNING AND REASONING

1. How do the historical presence of occupational therapy and the current practice of mental health occupational therapy mirror each other when working with the mental health population?

2. Why is it important to consider client interests, especially with this population, when planning evaluation and treatment interventions? Consider here the importance of "motivation" as this enhances participation.

3. On the basis of your own interests, identify two or three activities in which you regularly participate. Determine exactly what you get out of your participation and how you feel after your participation. The same things apply to your clients.

4. Using one current event issue from the media, determine how the mental health of another person or a group of people is being portrayed and reported. Is this an accurate representation of mental health problems or a case of a "media blitz" of information? Consider issues such as gun control, school shootings, suicide, or suicide attempts by well-known people, for example. Keep in mind that the ways mental health issues are presented affect how the overall population responds and develops beliefs and perspectives.

REFERENCES

Accordino, M., Porter, D. & Morse, L. (2001). Deinstitutionalization of persons with severe mental illness: Context and consequences. *The Journal of Rehabilitation, 67*, 2.

Allen, C.K., Austin, S.L., Earhart, C.A., McCrath, D.B., & Riska, W.L. (2007). Manual for the Allen Cognitive Level Screen (ACLS) and Large Allen Cognitive Level Screen. Caramito, CA: ACLS and LACLS Committee.

American Occupational Therapy Association, (2014). Fact Sheet: OT's Role in Community Mental Health. Retrieved from: http:www.aota.org

American Occupational Therapy Foundation. (2006). *AOTA's Centennial Vision.* Retrieved from https://www.aota.org/-/media/corporate/files/aboutaota/centennial/background/vision1.pdf

American Psychiatric Association. (2004). *Diagnostic and statistical manual of mental disorders* (4th ed., text revision). Washington, DC: Author.

American Psychiatric Association. (2013). *Diagnostic and statistical manual of mental disorders* (5th ed.). Washington, DC: Author.

Black, M.M. (1976) Adolescent role assessment. *American Journal of Occupational Therapy, 30*, 2, 73-79.

Bonder, B. (2015). *Psychosocial occupational therapy* (5th ed.). Thorofare, NJ: SLACK Incorporated.

Brown, C., & Dunn, W. (2002) *Adolescent and Adult Sensory Profile.* New York, NY: Pearson.

Bullock, A., & Bannigan, K. (2011). Effectiveness of activity-based group work in community mental health: A systematic review. *American Journal of Occupational Therapy, 65*, 257-266.

Canadian Association of Occupational Therapy. (1992). *The Canadian Occupational Performance Measure.* Toronto, CA: Author.

Cole, M. (2012). *Group dynamics in psychosocial occupational therapy.* Thorofare, NJ: SLACK Incorporated.

Creek, J. (2003). *Occupational Therapy and Mental Health Skills: Principles and Practice.* Churchill Livingstone: London.

D'Amico, M., Jaffee, L., & Gibson, R. (2010). Mental health evidence in the *American Journal of Occupational Therapy. American Journal of Occupational Therapy, 64*, 660-669.

Denten, . (1987). Psychiatric occupational therapy: A workbook of practical skills. Ch. 3. Little, Brown: Boston, MA.

Dunn, W. (1999). *The Sensory Profile.* New York, NY: Pearson.

Edelsen, J. (1996). *Lorna Jean King: A tribute to Lorna Jean King.* Retrieved from www.devdelay.org/newsletter/articles/pdf/2

Gutman, S. (2011). Special issue: Effectiveness of occupational therapy services in mental health practice. *American Journal of Occupational Therapy, 65*, 235-237.

Gutman, S. (2012). State of mental health in the American Journal of Occupational Therapy, 2008–2011. *American Journal of Occupational Therapy, 66*, e30-e33.

Hughes, J. (1996). *Organization and information at the bed-side: The experience of the medical division of labor by university hospital inpatients.* Department of Sociology, University of Chicago. Nov 1994. Retrieved from: http://www.changesurfer.com

Katz, N.,Bar-Haim, E., Livni, L. & Averback, S. (2012). Dynamic lowenstein occupational therapy cognitive assessment: Evaluation of potential to change in cognitive performance. American *Journal of Occupational Therapy, 66*, 2, 207-214.

Kohlman, L. (1992). *The Kohlman Evaluation of Living Skills (KELS),* 3rd. ed. American Occupational Therapy Association: Rockville, MD.

Itzkovick, M., Elazher, B., & Katz, N. (1996). *The Lowenstein Occupational Therapy Cognitive Assessment.* Morgan Hill, CA: North Coast Medical and Rehabilitation Products.

Matsutsuyu, J.S. (1969). The interest checklist. *American Journal of Occupational Therapy.* 23, 323-328.

Medley-Rath, S. (2012). The Sick Role Conflict. Sociology in Focus. Retrieved from: http://sociology-infocus.com/2012/12/the-sick-role-conflict/

Mini-Mental State Examination (1975). Mini-Mental State Examination: A practical method for grading the cognitive status of patients test for clinicians. *Journal of Psychiatric Research*, 12, 189-198.

Renoir, T., Hasebe, K., & Gray, L. (2013). Mind and body: How the health of the body impacts on neuropsychiatry. *Frontiers in Pharmacology, 4*, 158.

Schropler, E., & Bourgondien, M. (2010). *The Childhood Autism Rating Scale* (2nd ed.). Torrance, CA: Western Psychological Services.

Stiggelbout, A., and Kiebert, G.M. (1997). A role for the sick role: Patient preferences regarding information and practice in clinical decision making. *CMAJ,* 157 4, 383-389.

Substance Abuse and Mental Health Service Administration. (n.d.). *SAMHSA-HRSA Center for Integrated Health Solutions.* Retrieved from https://www.integration.samhsa.gov/

Williams, S., & Bloomer, J. (n.d.). *The Bay Area Functional Performance Evaluation.* Pequannock, NJ: Maddack. Retrieved from: http://www.maddak.com/bafpe-bay-area-functional-performance-evaluation-p-27817.html

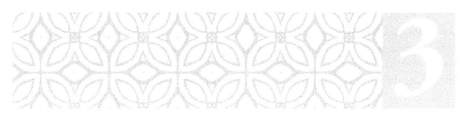

Practice in the
Physical Disability Arena

KEY WORDS

- Activities of daily living (ADL)
- Adaptive equipment
- Arthritis
- Cardiac problems
- Cerebrovascular accident (CVA)
- Diabetes
- Habilitation
- Multiple sclerosis (MS)
- Neurological conditions
- Orthopedic concerns
- Osteoarthritis (OA)
- Parkinson's disease (PD)
- Rehabilitation
- Rheumatoid arthritis (RA)
- Sexuality and sexual activity
- Spinal cord injury (SCI)
- Splinting
- Traumatic brain injury (TBI)

Hattjar, B.
Fundamentals of Occupational Therapy:
An Introduction to the Profession (pp. 33-58).
© 2019 Taylor & Francis Group.

The physical disabilities area of occupational therapy is broad and includes a variety of diagnoses consisting of diseases, illness, and injuries. The intent of this chapter is to provide students with basic information about a work arena in which occupational therapists regularly participate. This chapter is not an exhaustive review of all the physical disability diagnoses with which occupational therapists work, however.

HISTORY

Occupational therapists began to expand their clinical scope during World War I. At that time, therapists, then referred to as *reconstruction aides* (see Chapter 1), worked with soldiers who had been injured in the war. It is important to note that World War I was a "ground war." This means that the war was literally fought on land; guns, shells, tanks, and ammunition items were the tools of war. The types of injuries that were encountered by treating therapists include the following:

- Shrapnel (metal fragments which pierced or cut the skin)
- Bullet wounds
- Injuries sustained from grenade explosions
- Bayonet injuries (the sharp piercing terminal device of a rifle; similar to a knife wound)
- Traumatic injuries to the extremities, including amputation or loss of part of a limb (Box 3-1)

The roles and responsibilities of the reconstruction aides expanded due to the large number of soldiers who were injured. Interventions in the area of physical injuries, illnesses, and disabilities moved the fledgling profession from "invalid" or bedside activities to more general and diverse physical disability practice.

The reconstruction aides received accolades for their work with soldiers—so much so, that they began to be used in veterans hospitals immediately after the war. The positive news spread to the private sector, and occupational therapists began to expand their work domain to include private hospitals, clinics, and facilities. This growth and continued work with physical disabilities continued throughout the second and third decades of the 20th century. During the Second World War, occupational therapists were again utilized to work with soldiers who sustained battle-related injuries. During this war, injuries resulted from bullets, grenades, bomb explosions, burns, and fatigue (where injuries occurred due to limited rest and great exertion—hence, decreased reaction time, safety awareness, etc.; frequently referred to as *battle fatigue*).

After World War II, occupational therapists expanded their client base to include work with children and youth, adolescents, adults, and older people who sustained a variety of physical injuries, illnesses, or related disabilities.

To meet the growing demand for occupational therapists and to address the limited number of educational training programs for the 4-year, bachelor degree entry point into the profession, 2-year technical programs were developed in the late 1950s and early 1960s. This associate degree program entitled the graduates to use the title

---

Box 3-1

War-Related Limb Loss

World War I saw the introduction of wound-healing protocols. Because of improved wound-healing protocols, infection or subsequent death were less certain than during the Civil War when amputation or a severe wound occurred. The technique of delayed primary wound closure was instituted (Millard, 1986). This technique involves application of wet-to-dry dressing application over the involved area for approximately 2 to 3 days, followed by wound-suturing (sewing closed) via stitches in approximately 3 to 4 days. This technique saved lives and reduced the spread of infections when used correctly and consistently.

Box 3-2

Quality of Life and Health-Related Quality of Life

QOL is defined as something that "measures the difference, at a particular moment in time, between the hopes and expectations of the individual and that individual's present experiences" (Calman, 1984, p. 1250). A person's QOL is affected by age, sex, circumstance(s), health status, economic status, social and emotional status, and personal perception of life and life in general. As a profession, occupational therapy seeks to improve a client's QOL by considering the individual holistically as a whole, dynamic being in regard to his or her occupational responsibilities, roles, strengths, and limitations.

Health-related QOL (HRQoL; Healthy People 2020) expands on the QOL concept. HRQoL is a multidimensional concept that relates to physical, mental, emotional, and social functioning. HRQoL also seeks to determine clients satisfaction with his or her personal health, health care, and sense of well-being. Healthy People 2020 is a federal endeavor sponsored by the U.S. Department of Health and Human Services and focuses on client outcomes, client well-being, and the effect of health on social participation within cultural bounds.

---

of certified occupational therapy assistant (COTA). COTAs worked with the supervision and guidance of a registered occupational therapist (OTR). With both the OTR and COTA levels of practice, the profession was able to meet the individuals' needs more readily, and the profession continued to flourish.

Throughout the 1960s and 1970s, occupational therapy personnel expanded their domain of practice into more focused upper extremity evaluation and treatment, technology (including low-tech items such as seating systems or cushions for wheelchairs, custom *splinting* to maintain function or to prevent further loss of function or deformity), work with children who had physical disabilities, work-related injuries and cumulative trauma injuries, more intensive work with older people in nursing homes or hospital rehabilitation units, and introduction of concepts of safety and quality of life (QOL) into therapy (Box 3-2).

Box 3-3

RECERTIFICATION DOCUMENTATION

The recertification process for Medicare clients (also called the *plan of care*) is usually completed every 30 days on a specific form identified by Medicare. This form includes information about the client's diagnosis, long- and short-term treatment goals, and goal attainment or revisions made during the previous 30 days; it also must clearly identify the goals for the next 30-day period. To receive Medicare approval for continued care of the client, there must be both proof of need and proof of progress on identified goals. The recertification process need not be a lengthy review of the client's status but should include goals that are measurable, observable, and objective. A clear time frame— that is, the number of visits that are being requested—must also be indicated. This form is reviewed by Medicare billing, and notification of approval or rejection of the recertification request is provided by Medicare reviewers.

The 1980s saw the development and institution of Diagnosis-Related Groups (DRGs), which classifies a patient's hospital stay into various groups to facilitate payment of services. DRGs are based on a patient's average length of stay in hospitals and related facilities. Under this system, the health care system experienced a significant decrease in the number of "insurance-billable" days that could be reimbursed at a specific level of care. The most rigorous level of care was determined to be that in hospitals. A client, after achieving the maximum hospital length of stay, could be referred to a lesser level of care, for example, to outpatient care, home care, or nursing home care. This created new health care arenas for occupational therapist employment. It also necessitated greater efficiency and timeliness in the evaluation and treatment interventions by all health care professionals, including occupational therapists.

In 1998, capitation on Medicare and Medicare billing or charges was passed by our government. This was done to stop "overbilling" and high charges for Medicare recipients and to limit or stop charges for testing or interventions deemed unnecessary or excessive, or those that were duplicated by different health care providers. In much the same way that DRGs affected hospital length of stay, capitation, related to billable charges per year, permitted occupational therapists to bill a maximum of $1,500 per year per client for Medicare, the major source of health care insurance for people aged 65 years and older. This limited the number of client billable services a therapist could perform unless the therapist requested additional visits in a recertification process or in a "letter of medical necessity" (Box 3-3). However, even with a letter of medical necessity, there was still a $1,500 charge capitation on service reimbursement (Box 3-4).

This process creates additional work for therapists, so it is important to become proficient at writing these letters. Being able to write effective letters of medical necessity can also be helpful in situations in which an insurance company must approve additional occupational therapy client visits.

Box 3-4

LETTER OF MEDICAL NECESSITY

The ability to write an effective letter of medical necessity is a skill you will need to master as an occupational therapist. Always remember to be clear and concise and to maintain a positive demeanor in your writing. The letter should include the following:

1. State who you are, how long you have known the client, and the service you are requesting (in this case, occupational therapy).

2. Explain why the service you are requesting is necessary for the client.

3. Use support statements from the medical chart and/or your records and progress notes. It is not your judgment but the client's ability to make progress, based on your treatment, that constitutes medical necessity.

4. Expand on your statements to provide more evidence that what you are requesting will make a positive difference in the client's functional status.

5. Provide specific information including, but not limited to, how your treatments will prevent illness or disability or client decline that would require more assistance in the future. Explain how your treatments will assist the client in maintaining his or her functional abilities/capacity. Explain how your treatments will ameliorate the physical, mental, or developmental effects of the client's illness, injury, or disability.

6. Provide examples of specific data that may be helpful (e.g., how the client responded, interventions you have tried, the results your interventions have attained).

7. Always end your letter by stating what you believe will result if your request is not approved.

Note: If you are requesting durable medical equipment (DME) for the client, always check the manufacturer's website or, if it is Medicare you are dealing with, check the Medicare website for client needs specifics (PA Health Law Project, 2014). Reimbursement may be specific to the clients medical insurance. DME includes, but is not limited to, items such as hospital beds, portable toilets, a wheelchair or a walker, for example. Note that equipment such as raised toilet seats, shower chairs, grab bars, adjustable showerheads, and other bathroom items are not covered under Medicare.

Because of the increasing number of people over age 50 years in the United States, the baby boomers, the need for therapy services has increased and is expected to increase further during the first part of the 21st century (see Chapter 1, Box 1-3).

Chronic conditions such as heart disease, stroke (*cerebrovascular accident* [CVA]), *diabetes*, and *arthritis* are some of the most common, costly, and preventable health issues affecting Americans today (Centers for Disease Control and Prevention [CDC], cited by DeRosa, 2013). The paradigm shift from treatment of acute diagnoses to chronic conditions is expected to continue creating additional challenges for the U.S. health care system (DeRosa, 2013).

The first decade of the 21st century saw an increase in patient deductibles for insurance (the amount paid out of pocket paid upfront before insurance "kicks in" for service payment). Also, therapists needed to become increasingly productive and prudent in their provision of services to ensure profit and stability in their places of employment. The health care arena has become a more businesslike setting than ever before, and the therapist must be aware of this. It is unclear how health care will evolve, but one thing is certain: it will change. The Affordable Care Act (ACA) is currently being tested, reviewed, and expanded upon in order to be more inclusive. Nevertheless, opponents of health care changes want to repeal this act for a variety of reasons. The results of the status of health care accessibility and affordability in the United States remain to be finalized. This will affect how therapy services are provided and to what extent they will remain billable or reimbursable for service providers. It is up to the therapist to remain politically aware of all health care and insurance reimbursement changes. It is valuable for professionals in the field to support state and national political action committees (PACs), which are subcommittees of the national and state occupational therapy organizations. PACs use political lobbyists in state and federal government to promote causes and laws that align with the occupational therapy profession and assist in maintaining the domain of practice. PACs rely on the contribution of therapist members for funding. Please review Chapter 1, Box 1-3 for the names and dates of generations in the United States.

PRACTICE IN THE PHYSICAL DISABILITY ARENA

Occupational therapists who work with clients with disabilities must have a strong knowledge base of a variety of diagnoses, assessments, interventions, and *adaptive equipment*. In the realm of physical disabilities, we work with both *rehabilitation* (i.e., assisting clients in relearning skills and actions that have been lost due to an illness, injury, or disability) and *habilitation* (i.e., helping clients learn something for the first time or in a very different manner—how to perform an action or assigned role or to make accommodations in various real-world situations with a disability). In simple terms, we help our clients learn or relearn how to navigate their life in the presence of a physical disability. We help our clients to remain occupationally engaged beings.

COMMON DIAGNOSES

To provide a general overview of the most common types of diagnosis groups with whom occupational therapists work, the following diagnosis groups are reviewed:
- Endocrine problems
- Arthritis
- *Neurological conditions*
- *Cardiac problems*
- *Orthopedic concerns*

Endocrine Problems

The endocrine system comprises "those organs, or tissues within organs, that secrete their cellular products into the bloodstream rather than into the viscera (organs), cavities, or outside the body" (Hart & Loeffler, 2012, p. 379). The endocrine

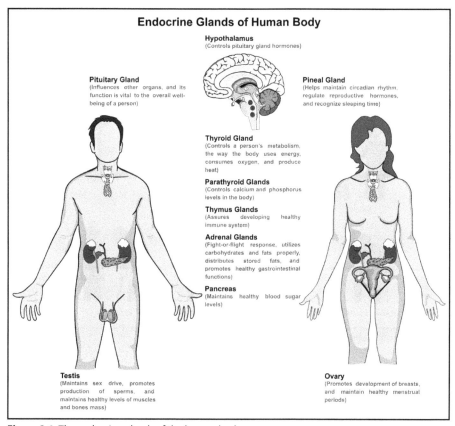

Figure 3-1. The endocrine glands of the human body.

system includes the glands in the body (Figure 3-1), and any problems with a gland can affect energy, growth, food utilization, maintenance of blood glucose levels, hormone levels, and a variety of other functions necessary for health and wellness. Depending on the endocrine problem, the occupational therapist may deal with energy conservation (in hypothyroidism), stress and anxiety reduction (in hyperthyroidism), self-care and *activities of daily living* (ADL), diabetes (which affects the pancreas), amputations (in diabetes, a limb may be amputated because of poor circulation or infection, resulting necrosis or death of the tissue), vision (eye problems in diabetes), and a wide variety of other physical and psychological issues.

With any endocrine system problem, ensuring that the client is capable of performing daily occupations and is able to assume occupational roles is a major concern. Many times, endocrine problems are diagnosed secondarily to some other problem. In this case, the primary diagnosis is the treatment focus, but the therapist must also carefully include and consider secondary endocrine problems in treatment. Additionally, the introduction of appropriate medications to combat the endocrine

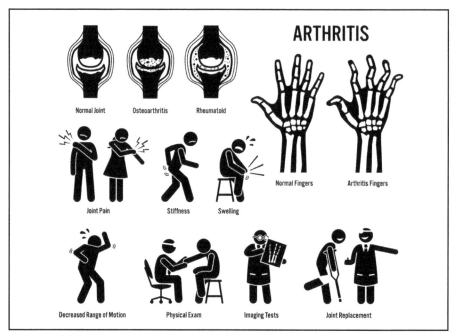

Figure 3-2. Visual representations of arthritis.

problem will often result in a decrease of symptoms, so medication management is an important consideration.

Arthritis

The word arthritis can be defined by its syllables: *arthro* refers to a joint, and *itis* refers to inflammation (Figure 3-2). Therefore, arthritis is an inflammation of a joint or joints (CDC, 2014a). When multiple joints are affected by arthritis, it is referred to as *polyarthritis*—many (*poly*) inflamed joints. Arthritis is divided into two distinct types: *osteoarthritis* (OA) and *rheumatoid arthritis* (RA). OA is also known as *degenerative joint disease* and is associated with the aging process. By age 65 years, 49.7% of people are diagnosed with OA. It is most prevalent in the weightbearing joints of the legs and hips, ankles, and low back. OA is also diagnosed in the neck or cervical area of the spine. Generally, OA is accompanied with outward visible signs of joint changes.

RA is an autoimmune disease in which the body attacks itself, most commonly in the synovium (or synovial fluid area) of the joints. It is accompanied by physical symptoms of fatigue, a general feeling of not being well (malaise), a persistent aching of the joints, and visible joint changes. Frequently, the occupational therapist is called on to fabricate splints for hands and wrists and to educate the client in correct performance of daily activities to avoid excessive stress on the joint. Also included in this intervention is education and training in correct body mechanics, work simplification, and joint protection (Box 3-5).

Box 3-5

BODY MECHANICS, WORK SIMPLIFICATION, AND JOINT PROTECTION

BODY MECHANICS

Body mechanics is a term used to described the manner in which the body is used to accomplish a variety of tasks, including: tasks associated with moving or transferring clients; moving items at work (e.g., boxes, tools, or equipment); carrying or moving infants or children at home, in transit, or in treatment; and performing routine daily tasks such as food preparation, bathing, grooming, and dressing, as determined by the occupation an individual encounters throughout the day. Body mechanics relates to both the professionals and the clients. The therapist should demonstrate correct body mechanics for the client, and the client should demonstrate understanding by "doing" the movement correctly. The following are basic percepts of good body mechanics:

- Keep a stable center of gravity (COG) in relation to what is being moved. Your COG is located at approximately your belly button or right below your waist level at midline body orientation. The closer a weight load is to your COG, the easier that weight will be controlled and moved, so weight or "loads" should be kept as close to the COG as possible. Conversely, the farther an object is placed from the COG, the more difficult it is to control, and the greater the force shears or weight will be. The heavier the weight the body experiences, the more difficult it is to retain good body mechanics and safety.

- Maintain a wider base of support to ensure balance and stability (with legs approximately shoulder width apart and body weight equally distributed, resulting in a symmetrical body position).

- Bend and lift or move items with your legs, hips, and thighs, not your lower back. Most low back injuries occur at the lumbar level (L 4-5) due to poor lifting or object management. In accordance with this, lift with your arms, legs, and your body force. The larger muscles of the legs and arms are more resilient and stronger than the small muscles surrounding the spine, which are not designed to move heavy objects, but to keep the spine in alignment and symmetrical.

- Keep the body in a symmetrical and aligned position and do not twist, turn, or torque the body (Sladyk et al., 2010) when moving weight. Twisting, turning, and torque compromise the body and increase the likelihood of injury.

WORK SIMPLIFICATION

Work simplification means keep work as simple as possible to decrease body stress and the likelihood of injury or fatigue. Some basic principles of work simplification follow:

- Sit rather than stand if possible while doing work tasks.

- Maintain a directional "flow" or direction for work activities at the tabletop or desk. If your are right-hand dominant, things should flow from left to right; if you are left-handed, things should flow from right to left in most situations (including activities such as desk or tabletop work, or even washing and rinsing dishes).

- Plan and structure work tasks. Perform things that are more difficult and energy exerting first, then perform things that are easier and less stressful.

- Break work tasks down into reasonable parts or components, rather than trying to complete everything all at once. This decreases emotional stress and physiological stressors such as high blood pressure or joint stress. Tasks can be broken down into smaller components to permit a short break between work task sequences.

(continued)

> # Box 3-5 (CONTINUED)
>
> ## Body Mechanics, Work Simplification, and Joint Protection
>
> - If possible, slide objects over a flat surface rather than lifting the objects. Additionally, try to decrease the force or "drag" by placing objects to be moved on friction-decreasing flat, smooth surfaces or by using carts with wheels to move or transport.
> - Push rather than pull because this is less stressful on the body.
> - Take breaks and stretch to avoid fatigue, excessive joint pain, or joint discomfort.
> - Always consider how tasks can be broken down into segments or steps to accommodate potential fatigue or joint stress or pain. In other words, "think before you move."
>
> ### JOINT PROTECTION
>
> These simple techniques decrease joint stress and fatigue:
> - Keep the wrists in a neutral position as opposed to having the wrists in flexion or extension for long periods of time.
> - Perform gentle stretches during brief stretch breaks if activities are of a long duration.
> - Avoid ulnar deviation of wrists for activities; this is a detrimental and deforming position.
> - Avoid excessive and repetitive grasp or pinch of objects because this promotes joint deformity over time.

Other types of arthritis or diseases associated with an arthritic component include fibromyalgia, a symmetrical (equal on both sides of the body) pattern of pain and discomfort located throughout the body; juvenile RA, with onset in children and youth; and gouty arthritis (Box 3-6), a painful form usually seen in the great toe and associated with high uric acid levels and a rich, fatty diet. However, there are more than 100 types of arthritis (CDC, 2014a; Sladyk, Jacobs, & MacRae, 2010).

Arthritis is usually accompanied by pain, achiness, crepitus (i.e., creaking or crunching) at a specific joint, along with a decreased active range of motion at the involved joint(s). Clients frequently report that they can easily detect a change in the weather (actually the barometric pressure) in their arthritic joints because their symptoms increase or there is the presence of persistent joint discomfort. Arthritic patients are subject to increased symptoms when the weather changes from warm to cool (autumn) and cool to warm (spring). Humidity levels also seem to affect arthritic symptoms. Once weather stabilizes, weather-associated pain or discomfort also decreases in arthritis patients.

Some arthritis patients respond better to cryotherapy (cold), whereas others respond well to neutral warmth or heat. Medication also is helpful to these patients; common medications prescribed for arthritis patients include over-the-counter ibuprofen, acetaminophen, and aspirin or derivatives of these. Additionally, many prescription-only medications exist that decrease the pain and persistence of this disease. As pain levels decrease and range of motion and function improve, these

Box 3-6

Benjamin Franklin and the Gout

Benjamin Franklin (1706-1790)

Midnight, 22 October, 1780

FRANKLIN. Eh! Oh! Eh! What have I done to merit these cruel sufferings?

GOUT. Many things; you have ate and drank too freely, and too much indulged those legs of yours in their indolence.

FRANKLIN. Who is it that accuses me?

GOUT. It is I, even I, the Gout.

FRANKLIN. What! My enemy in person?

GOUT. No, not your enemy.

FRANKLIN. I repeat it; my enemy; for you would not only torment my body to death, but ruin my good name; you reproach me as a glutton and a tippler; now all the world, that knows me, will allow that I am neither the one nor the other.

GOUT. The world may think as it pleases; it is always very complaisant to itself, and sometimes to its friends; but I very well know that the quantity of meat and drink proper for a man who takes a reasonable degree of exercise, would be too much for another, who never takes any.

FRANKLIN. I take-Eh! Oh!-as much exercise-Eh!-as I can, Madam Gout. You know my sedentary state, and on that account, it would seem, Madam Gout, as if you might spare me a little, seeing it is not altogether my own fault.

GOUT. Not a jot; your rhetoric and your politeness are thrown away; your apology avails nothing. You ought to walk or ride; or, if the weather prevents that, play at billiards. But let us examine your course of life. While the mornings are long, and you have leisure to go abroad, what do you do? Why, instead of gaining an appetite for breakfast, by salutary-exercise, you amuse yourself with books, pamphlets, or newspapers, which commonly are not worth the reading. Yet you eat an inordinate breakfast, four dishes of tea, with cream, and one or two buttered toasts, with slices of hung beef. What is your practice after dinner? Walking in the beautiful gardens of those friends, with whom you have dined, would be the choice of men of sense; but these are rejected for this abominable game of chess. But amidst my instructions, I had almost forgot to administer my wholesome corrections; so take that twinge,—and that.

FRANKLIN. Oh! Eh! Oh! Ohhh! As much instruction as you please, Madam Gout, and as many reproaches; but pray, Madam, a truce with your corrections!

GOUT. No, Sir, no,—I will not abate a particle of what is so much for your good,—therefore—

FRANKLIN. Your reasonings grow very tiresome.

GOUT. I stand corrected. I will be silent and continue my office; take that, and that.

FRANKLIN. Oh I Ohh! Talk on, I pray you!

GOUT. No, no; I have a good number of twinges for you to-night, and you may be sure of some more to-morrow.

FRANKLIN. What, with such a fever! I shall go distracted. Oh! Eh! Can no one bear it for me?

GOUT. Ask that of your horses; they have served you faithfully.

FRANKLIN. How can you so cruelly sport with my torments?

(continued)

BOX 3-6 (CONTINUED)

BENJAMIN FRANKLIN AND THE GOUT

GOUT. Sport! I am very serious. I have here a list of offences against your own health distinctly written, and can justify every stroke inflicted on you.

FRANKLIN. Read it then.

GOUT. It is too long a detail; but I will briefly mention some particulars.

FRANKLIN. Proceed. I am all attention.

GOUT. Do you remember how often you have promised yourself, the following morning, a walk in the grove, or in your own garden, and have violated your promise, alleging, at one time it was too cold, at another too warm, too windy, too moist, or what else you pleased; when in truth it was too nothing but your insuperable love of ease?

FRANKLIN. That I confess may have happened occasionally, probably ten times in a year.

GOUT. Your confession is very far short of the truth; the gross amount is one hundred and ninety-nine times...

FRANKLIN. I am convinced now of the justness of poor Richard's remark, that "Our debts and our sins are always greater than we think for."

GOUT. So it is. You philosophers are sages in your maxims, and fools in your conduct.

FRANKLIN. But do you charge, among my crimes, that I return in a carriage from Mr. Brillon's?

GOUT. Certainly; for having been seated all the while, you cannot object the fatigue of the day, and cannot want, therefore, the relief of a carriage.

FRANKLIN. What, then, would you have me do with my carriage?

GOUT. Burn it, if you choose; you would at least get heat out of it once in this way; or, if you dislike that proposal, here's another for you; observe the poor peasants, who work in the vineyards and grounds about the villages; you may find every day, among these deserving creatures, four or five old men and women, bent and perhaps crippled by weight of years and too long and too great labor. After a most fatiguing day, these people have to trudge a mile or two to their smoky huts. Order your coachman to set them down. This is an act that will be good for your soul; and, at the same time, after your visit to the Brillons, if you return on foot, that will be good for your body.

FRANKLIN. Ah! how tiresome you are!

GOUT. Well, then, to my office; it should not be forgotten that I am your physician. There.

FRANKLIN. Ohhh! what a devil of a physician!

GOUT. How ungrateful you are to say so!

FRANKLIN. I never feed physician or quack of any kind, to enter the list against you; if, then, you do not leave me to my repose, it may be said you are ungrateful too.

GOUT. I can scarcely acknowledge that as any objection. As to quacks, I despise them; they may kill you indeed, but cannot injure me. there.

FRANKLIN. Oh! Oh!—for Heaven's sake leave me; and I promise faithfully never more to play at chess, but to take exercise daily, and live temperately.

GOUT. I know you too well. You promise fair; but after a few months of good health, you will return to your old habits; your fine promises will be forgotten like the forms of the last year's clouds. Let us then finish the account, and I will go. But I leave you with an assurance of visiting you again at a proper time and place..

Reprinted from Matthews, 1914.

patients usually experience a good prognosis for a period of time. The exception to this is RA, which is characterized by periods of exacerbations (symptom increase) and remissions (symptom decreases). RA may be accompanied by a general sense of malaise or aches and pains.

Some clients prefer to use homeopathic or naturopathic medications. These must be reported, especially if the client is using both homeopathic and traditional Western medicine, because negative interactions may occur. Some patients indicate that they experience common gastrointestinal discomfort associated with arthritis medications, especially if these medications are used over a lengthy period of time, and instead opt for homeopathic medication. Homeopathic medications tend to take longer to produce a positive effect—generally 10 to 21 days.

Neurological Conditions

Perhaps the most commonly seen diagnosis groups seen by occupational therapists among neurological conditions is a CVA, commonly referred to as a *stroke*. CVAs can be *hemorrhagic* (i.e., a "bleed" into the brain caused by a blood vessel rupturing) or *ischemic* (i.e., blood flow is cut off by a blood clot, resulting in tissue necrosis or death; Gould & Dyer, 2011). The area(s) of the brain affected and the side of the brain where the insult occurred determine the deficits the client will experience. If a CVA occurs on the right side of the brain, the left side of the body will be affected and vice versa (due to the corpus callosum or brain crossover area).

Other neurological conditions seen in occupational therapy include *Parkinson's disease* (PD), *multiple sclerosis* (MS), *traumatic brain injury* (TBI), and *spinal cord injury* (SCI), among many other diagnoses.

In PD, certain nerve cells in the brain gradually break down or die. Symptoms of the disease include distal hand tremors, slow movement (bradykinesia), muscle rigidity, impaired balance and posture, loss of automatic movements (blinking the eyes, swinging the arms when walking, facial gestures, smiling or frowning), changes in speech or speech slurring, difficulty writing, and decreased proprioception. These symptoms are caused by a loss of nerve cells or neurons that produce dopamine, a chemical in the brain that acts as a messenger from the brain to the body, especially the muscles and joints. When dopamine levels decrease, abnormal brain activity occurs, and this results in PD (Mayo Clinic, 2014). PD is most prevalent in older men, although younger men (e.g., actor Michael J. Fox) have been diagnosed early in their fourth decade of life. Michael J. Fox, an award winning Canadian actor, was diagnosed with early-onset PD in 1988 at the age of approximately 30 years old. He has continued to work as an actor and founded the Michael J. Fox Foundation for Parkinson's Research (Michael J. Fox Foundation, 2018).

MS involves an immune-mediated process in which the body's immune system is directed against the central nervous system, which includes the brain, spinal cord, and optic nerves. The body's immune system attacks the myelin sheath that surrounds the nerves, resulting in the development of sclerotic plaques. This disrupts the nerve conduction mechanism to and from the brain and spinal cord, and a variety of symptoms result (National Multiple Sclerosis Society, 2018). (It may be helpful to think about this myelin sheath destruction as a frayed electric cord to better visualize the process.) The resulting symptoms may seem unrelated, inconsistent, or not disease-oriented, and MS may be mild, moderate, or severe in its course. It is characterized by periods of remission, when symptoms decrease or disappear, and periods of symptom exacerbation. This makes daily occupations and planning for the future a difficult process for these clients. MS is most often diagnosed in blonde, blue-eyed women of northern or Scandinavian cultures (it is two to three times more common in women than men; National Multiple Sclerosis Society, 2018), and the diagnosis is made during the third or fourth decade of life. The incidence of this disease decreases substantially as one gets closer to the equator and warmer climates. In some tropical cultures, the incidence of MS is quite low or almost unheard of.

A TBI is caused by a bump, blow, or jolt to the head or a penetrating head injury that disrupts the normal function of the brain. The symptoms of a TBI can be mild, with a brief change or alteration of mental status or consciousness, to severe, in which a prolonged or extended period of coma or unconsciousness or amnesia occur after the head injury (CDC, 2014c). The common reasons for incurred TBIs include motor vehicle accidents, acts of violence, or accidental falls or blows to the head. In recent years, concussions have received significant media attention due to National Football League guidelines for concussion treatment and the increasing reports of retired or older players experiencing almost Alzheimer's-type dementia as they age. The use of alcohol or substances may also contribute to TBIs, in that the injury may occur during periods of altered consciousness.

An SCI may occur after damage to the spinal column. The spinal column comprises 31 bones called *vertebrae* (7 cervical vertebrae, 12 thoracic vertebrae, 5 lumbar vertebrae, 5 sacral vertebrae, and 2 fused coccyx vertebrae). The spinal cord, the central bundle of nerves extending from the brain and branching peripherally, is responsible for transmitting signals between the brain and the rest of the body. The cord is located within the spinal column. Any damage to the spinal column can affect the spinal cord and result in temporary or permanent neurological impairment. An SCI may result in paraplegia (the lower part of the body is paralyzed) or quadriplegia (paralysis from the injury sight and lower). The SCI may involve complete or incomplete severance of the spinal cord. In the case of an incomplete SCI, symptoms will vary depending on the site of the injury. SCI frequently occurs in younger males, and sexual functioning becomes an important issue for these people. The most common causes of SCIs include sporting or diving accidents, motor vehicle accidents, or accidents where alcohol or substances create altered judgment.

Cardiac Problems

Cardiac problems comprise a wide array of issues, including myocardial infarction (MI; commonly referred to as a *heart attack*), congestive heart failure (CHF), post-heart surgery clients, and clients diagnosed with heart rhythm problems (where the heart beats too slow, too fast, or a combination of slow and rapid beating), among other diagnoses. Occupational therapists work with clients who have cardiac conditions to help them attain independence and the ability to perform daily activities that are within their scope of ability. This includes ADL such as dressing, grooming, bathing, transferring, and functional ambulation, as well as *sexual activity*, which is an ADL that is not always addressed. ADL also include the performance of functional activities necessary for daily living at the client's level of ability, such as cooking, household management, child care or caregiving, and work-related tasks associated with employment or volunteering. It is important not to suggest activities that are too stressful on the heart nor those that offer no likelihood of building activity tolerance and endurance. Occupational therapists are frequently a part of the client's treatment team for these issues. The therapist must provide "just the right fit" for activities. It is important for the therapist to recognize signs of stress, including rapid and shallow breathing, perspiration, mouth breathing and lip pursing, and verbal reports of pain or discomfort while performing the activity. In the case of these signs of "overdoing," it is recommended that the client rest or take a short break from whatever task precipitated the event. This should also be reported to other health care staff and professionals. Most tasks require oxygen, pumped throughout the body, for performance. Breathing and oxygen flow oxygen is compromised in some cardiac patients. Fifty years ago or less, the major cause for cardiac problems resulted from familial or genetic tendencies or from cigarette smoking. Cardiac problems were much more common in men than women. However, in recent years, women have experienced an increase in cardiac problems, and stress-related issues are considered to be major contributor to this (Figure 3-3).

Common cardiac problems include the following:

- Bicuspid aortic valve defect: In this condition, the aortic valve has two, rather than three, cusps. It is manifested in adulthood and characterized by fatigue and heart murmur, accompanied by heart failure, in which the heart does not function optimally.
- Atrial and ventricular septal defects: In this embryonic anomaly, there is a hole in the septum between the right and left atria and/or a hole in the septum between the right and left ventricles. Symptoms include heart murmur, intolerance to exercise, and heart failure.
- Hypertrophic cardiomyopathy: This is an autosomal dominant mutation in which the interventricular septum is thickened. It can result in sudden death, arrhythmia, or infarction in the septum.
- Coarctation of the aorta: This embryonic anomaly results in stenosis of the descending aorta in the thorax. The femoral (lower extremity) pulse is weak, and the upper extremity evidences hypertension. A heart murmur is present, and heart failure usually results (Loeffler & Hart, 2015).
- CHF: This condition occurs when an enlarged heart can no longer pump blood throughout the body (Loeffler & Hart, 2015). In later stages, people with CHF appear bloated due to the buildup of fluid, cyanotic (blue in color) due to poor oxygenation of the blood throughout the body, and short of breath due to pulmonary edema.
- MI (or heart attack): An MI occurs when part of the heart is not functioning properly and the blood vessels that supply the heart become blocked, preventing

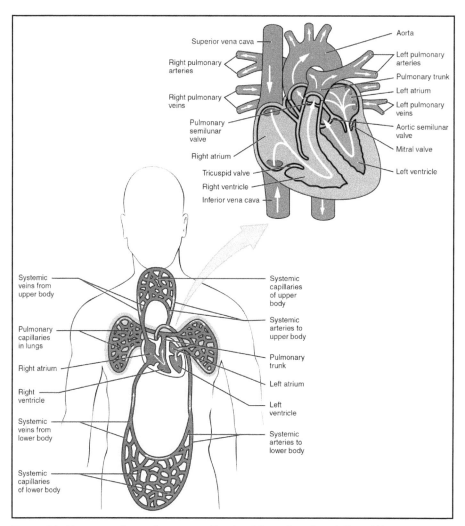

Figure 3-3. Human cardiovascular system. (Reprinted from OpenStax College (CC BY 3.0; http://creativecommons.org/licenses/by/3.0), via Wikimedia Commons.)

oxygen from getting to the heart. The heart, which is a muscle, either dies or becomes permanently damaged (Loeffler & Hart, 2015).

Orthopedic Concerns

Orthopedic concerns include joint articulation problems, postsurgery treatment (commonly for hip or knee replacements), osteoporosis, and postsurgery joint repair, among many other conditions. Orthopedic problems are usually associated with arthritis, past injury, or poor body mechanics throughout the life span and are associated with the aging process.

Box 3-7

HIP PRECAUTIONS AND USE OF ADAPTIVE EQUIPMENT FOR THE POSTSURGICAL HIP CLIENT

Hip precautions are directives that promote appropriate and correct healing of the postsurgical hip. The following are usually considered to be appropriate precautions:

- Avoidance of hip flexion greater than 90 degrees
- Avoidance of internal and external rotation of the hip joint
- Avoidance of hip hyperextension
- Sitting in a symmetrical position without leg crossing or ankle crossing
- Instruction to wear lower extremity compression garments to avoid blood clot formation or deep vein thrombosis. (This is not exclusive to hip surgery, but is a common postsurgical precaution.)
- Use of long-handle adaptive equipment for dressing and lower extremity bathing. (This usually includes a long shoehorn, a sock-donning aid, and a long-handle reacher. Such equipment decreases or eliminates the need to flex forward to dress the lower body.)

For postsurgical hip and knee clients, therapists work to maintain range of motion, ensure correct performance of ADL as a means to avoid compromised joint safety and integrity at the site of the surgery, educate and instruct the client in the use of adaptive equipment, and provide education for caregivers to ensure client safety and maintain alignment or integrity at the site of surgery. Caregivers must understand the rationale behind techniques the client will need to use daily (Box 3-7).

Depending on the nature of the orthopedic problem, rehabilitation for typical daily activities, occupations, and roles is a common intervention (e.g., rehabilitating a homemaker on body mechanics and joint positioning to perform cooking and kitchen activities) (see Box 3-5 on body mechanics, work simplification, and joint protection).

PRACTICE LOCATIONS

When working with clients who have physical disabilities, occupational therapists may practice in an acute setting, a long-term or skilled nursing unit of a hospital, a rehabilitation setting, in outpatient therapy, in a nursing home or assisted-living facility, or in home care. Practice in this area is usually dictated by the extent of clients' needs, their home situation, their age and skill level, and the type of diagnosis and limitations the clients have incurred.

WORK AS AN OCCUPATIONAL THERAPIST IN THE AREA OF PHYSICAL DISABILITIES

It is easy to surmise that a therapist working in the physical disability field must have knowledge of a wide variety of diagnoses, techniques, evaluations, and treatment skills. It is also important for the therapist who practices in this setting to be involved with continuing education to remain current with techniques and treatment modalities.

Screens and Evaluations

Many facilities use screens or evaluations that have been developed in-house; these types of assessments or screens vary greatly from facility to facility. However, the types of screens and assessments mentioned here are standardized (they must be done in a specific manner) and have been validated (the test results they yield are similar over time and in between evaluators). These types of tests or evaluations are considered reliable in that they test what they indicate they are testing.

Screens

A screen is a quick assessment of clients' ability to perform certain tasks, either physical in the case of disability or cognitive for psychosocial concerns (e.g., the Mini-Mental State Examination described in Chapter 2).

- Active Range of Motion Screen: A "mirrored" (the therapist sits directly across from the patient) display of active upper extremity range of motion at the neck, shoulder, elbow, forearm, wrist, and hand. The therapist asks the client to "do what I do as if you were looking in a mirror." Clients are asked to sit erect with their feet flat on the floor and to look at what the therapist does, then perform that movement or action with their arms. The movements included relate to the possible motion at the cervical and upper extremity joints and motion planes. The client is asked to "move to the point of pain or discomfort, not beyond." This brief screen gives the therapist a general idea of the amount of motion the client can accomplish independently. It is contraindicated for clients who are casted or splinted, have postsurgery stitches, or are not medically approved to perform particular movements actively or independently.

- ADL Screen: The client is asked to don and doff clothing such as their socks, an oversized shirt (put on over their clothing), and their shoes. This screen can be completed by the therapist or therapist assistant. Additionally, an occupational therapy assistant can complete the ADL aspect of the initial evaluation and report the findings back to the therapist. The intent is to determine whether the client has sufficient dexterity, range of motion, strength, endurance, and cognition to perform a common action. In the case of orthopedic clients, the use of adaptive equipment may be introduced to facilitate ADL involvement while eliminating joint compromise.

- Transfer Screen: Clients with poor balance, endurance, or motor planning can be asked to get up from their chair or bed, walk to a designated location (e.g., the bathroom in their hospital room or a window in the clinic) while the therapist observes and spots (to ensure safety) their movement. The client is then asked to return to the chair or bed and sit down. This type of functional ambulation is necessary for independent and safe living outside of the clinical setting. The use of adaptive equipment, such as a transfer board, may be introduced to facilitate transfer involvement while decreasing or eliminating any safety or balance issues.

If no problems are identified during the screening process, the client may not be a candidate for ongoing therapy. However, if problems are apparent during the screening process, these can be addressed in the evaluation and then in therapy interventions. It is important to remember that not everyone needs or meets the requirements for occupational therapy.

Evaluations

When clients exhibit obvious problems during the occupational therapy screen, they are usually recommended to receive an evaluation. The examples of evaluations provided in this chapter are not all inclusive and represent only a small portion of available evaluations in the occupational therapy profession. Those included here are those that are more commonly used, have undergone research, and have a good track record of reliability.

- Kohlman Evaluation Living Skills (KELS): The KELS Test Manual is designed to determine a person's ability to perform basic living skills (Kohlman Thompson, 1999). Although it was initially developed for use in the psychiatric setting, it has been generalized and is now used in many settings, including physical disabilities, in regard to living skill use in adult and older adult clients who desire to return home from a more intensive living situation. The KELS includes interview and observation components and is used primarily to determine the likelihood of safe, independent function in the community or for clients with psychiatric diagnoses or cognitive dysfunction (McGourtney, 1979).

- Functional Independence Measure (FIM): The FIM is widely used in a variety of clinical settings, including work with the physically disabled client population. The FIM uses a 7-point rating scale to describe the amount of assistance needed for the client to perform 18 tasks related to self-care, cognition, and communication. It can be used during the initial evaluation and as well as throughout treatment to determine client progress (increasing independence) or lack of progress (Uniform Data System for Medical Rehabilitation, 2000).

- The Assessment of Motor and Process Skills (AMPS): The AMPS includes 56 tasks typical to the instrumental ADL activities of children, adolescents, and adults to allow standardized ratings of specific motor and process skills (Fisher, 1999).

- The Canadian Occupational Performance Measure (COPM): The COPM is a highly client-centered assessment comprising a semistructured interview that helps clients identify their perception of occupational performance in the areas of self-care, leisure, and productivity (Law et al., 2005). This evaluation can be used during the initial evaluation and also during reevaluation sessions that occur throughout treatment. Topic areas, determined by the client with therapist input, are assessed in terms of task importance, satisfaction, and performance.

- The Occupational Self-Assessment (OSA): The OSA is a aligned with the Model of Human Occupation theory; it is a client self-report assessment that looks at clients' satisfaction with their performance on tasks and activities. The OSA also estimates clients' self-perception of task mastery (Kramer, Kielhofner, & Forsyth, 2012). It is quick and easy to administer.
- The Routine Task Inventory (RTI): Based on Claudia Allen's cognitive disability model, the RTI includes therapist-observed and client-reported self-care performance related to Allen's levels and modes of assistance required for a safe return to a lesser care environment such as the home (Heinmann, Allen, & Yerxa, 1989). To perform routine tasks safely, a client must have both cognitive and physical skills.
- Executive Function Performance Test (EFPT): Baum and test collaborators developed the EFPT to determine "what a person can do" in a performance-based, standardized assessment. This test assesses both performance of typical tasks and cognition (Baum, Monison, Hahn, & Edwards, 2003). With regard to this test, Baum states: "Functioning as a whole is examined as individuals perform an entire task." The purposes of this test are to determine (a) which executive functions are impaired, (b) an individual's capacity for independent functioning, and (c) the amount of assistance necessary for task completion. The EFPT uses four common and basic tasks that are considered "essential for self maintenance and independent living": cooking, telephone use, medication management, and bill payment. Cognitive components that this test includes are the components of task initiation (beginning the task), task execution (doing the task), sequencing (performing the task using the correct steps), judgment and safety (doing the task in an appropriate manner), and completion (finishing the task). By viewing the task in its entirety, appropriate recommendations can be made by the occupational therapist (Baum, Monison, Hahn, & Edwards, 2003).

Please note that many of these assessments or evaluations suggest that you carefully and considerately review the testing kit and testing manual. Most of these assessments suggest practice before actually performing them on a client. In other words, you must become familiar with the assessments before you use them in a clinical setting. This is an excellent piece of advice! Additionally, none of these evaluations are considered to be better or worse than any other. They are, however, frequently encountered in the clinical setting.

Treatment Interventions

As stated throughout this chapter, the scope of work in the physical disabilities area of occupational therapy is quite varied. Those who practice in this general area usually perform specific evaluations and therapeutic interventions based on the client diagnosis group with which they are working to meet client needs and address specific client issues and treatment intervention goals. The therapist would perform specific interventions related to the needs of the client. For example, on an orthopedic floor, the therapist might need to do more splinting, positioning, and self-care training, whereas on a neurological floor, the therapist might need to complete more self-care training to ensure safety, sequencing, and adherence to work techniques as might occur with cooking or daily self-care tasks such as showering. This may be translated into tabletop activities then come to fruition when the client has to incorporate some strategies learned into the actual performance of a task for home or self.

In reference to the diagnosis groups presented earlier in this chapter, treatment options might include, but not limited to, the following:

- Endocrine problems: When working with clients who experience problems with the endocrine system, intervention might include medication management, healthy food choices, healthy cooking and safe kitchen techniques (to avoid cuts or burns), skin or foot inspection techniques for diabetics, the selection of appropriate footwear and socks or stockings, maintenance of clean and healthy feet for diabetics, activity configuration assignments to account for times of high and low energy and the need for sleep (diabetics, thyroid, menopausal woman, and for women with menstrual irregularities), and so on.

- Arthritis: With the arthritic patient, pain or discomfort control or management is usually a primary focus and is accomplished with exercise, positioning, splinting, or passive or active movement. Concepts of work simplification, joint protection, and energy conservation are considered a prudent component for occupational therapy interventions with this client group. An activity configuration would also be helpful to determine times of higher or lower energy, thereby making time management and activity prioritization important.

- Neurological problems: This group includes diagnosis groups ranging from stroke (CVA), to PD, to MS. There are many other diseases in this category, but these three are typically seen by occupational therapists. With these diagnoses, a traumatic event occurs in the brain that disrupts messages sent from the brain to the spinal nerves. The results can be a devastating, including lack of voluntary motion in the body and difficulty with speech, mobility, and ADL. Other effects include diminished vision, swallowing and feeding problems, and cognitive changes. The maintenance of range of motion, strength, and task or activity endurance are important considerations for these clients, as are safety issues. The completion of daily self-care and household or work activities must be considered within the framework of therapy intervention. For many therapists, work with this client group includes the performance of a home evaluation if a return to the home is appropriate (Box 3-8).

- Cardiac problems: The type of cardiac problem dictates what occupational interventions will occur. For the post-MI client, resuming movement and reengagement in daily tasks safely is important, whereas transfer training with a postsurgical bypass patient would include transfer and positioning training to avoid undue pulling on postsurgical stitches while remaining mobile and performing typical daily tasks. These clients are also usually concerned with how the cardiac event will affect their personal life, especially in the area of *sexuality*.

BOX 3-8

HOME EVALUATION

A home evaluation occurs when a therapist goes to the client's home to assess safety threats, look at access in and out of the home, and see if spaces are sufficient to accommodate the client's status and any DME he or she may have. Many clients require the use of a hospital bed, a portable toilet, bathroom modifications, and safety tools (e.g., safety call buttons) to return to their home.

Frequently, cardiac patients are wary of resuming sexual activity for fear of precipitating another cardiac event (Box 3-9). In actuality, having sex and orgasm is no more stressful on the heart muscle and cardiovascular system than walking a short distance. It is important to have medical clearance from a physician before this intimate subject is broached and dealt with in occupational therapy (Hattjar, 2012) (Box 3-10).

- Orthopedic concerns: Generally, a client with orthopedic problems requires movement, instruction and education in safety techniques, symptom control due to discomfort or pain or postsurgery healing and recovery, positioning assistance, transfer training, and self-care training (ADL), and he or she also needs to increase endurance and strength to be functionally mobile. Specifically, the client might require training in ADL to retain the integrity of a surgery, as might occur with a hip or knee replacement. In many situations, clients may be wheelchair bound due to nonweightbearing status of a lower extremity, as might occur if a lower extremity bone is fractured or broken or after hip or knee replacement or surgery. In this type of situation, it is important to make sure that the client can move the wheelchair for functional activities (e.g., moving the wheelchair from one's room to the dining area, bathroom, etc.) or use other mobility aids such as a walker, quad cane (a cane that his a four-prong termination), single-prong cane, or even crutches. Both occupational and physical therapy may work on mobility. Once clients attain a partial weightbearing or toe-touch status, crutches or possibly a walker are used. This type of walking aid gets the client up from a seated position but requires arm strength—something that can be worked on with the wheelchair mobility tasks provided in anticipation of this. Depending on clients' physical status, pain level, and balance, they may graduate to the use of a quad cane. The intent of these functional mobility interventions is to resume occupational roles; regain of strength, range of motion, and endurance; improve safety awareness; promote adherence to safety precautions; and eventually enable the client to return to a lesser level of care or return to the home.

BOX 3-9

COMMON MYTHS ASSOCIATED WITH RESUMPTION OF SEXUAL ACTIVITY IN RELATION TO A PHYSICAL DISABILITY

Katz (2007) identified the following myths in regard to cardiac clients, but these items can be further generalized to include many of the diagnosis groups, with their own symptoms and peculiarities, as well:

- Myth 1: Sex is no longer permissible after a cardiac event such as an MI.
- Myth 2: Any person diagnosed with heart disease (or any physical disability) will experience chest pain (or some noxious symptom) during sexual activity.
- Myth 3: For older adults, sex is no longer important.

BOX 3-10

THE PLISSIT MODEL

The PLISSIT model (Annon, 1976) provides a logical structure and sequence for addressing the personal topic of sexuality with any client, including the cardiac client. PLISSIT is an acronym for

P: Permission

LI: Limited Information

SS: Specific Suggestions

IT: Intensive Therapy

CASE STUDY SCENARIOS

Arthritis

Mr. Jones resides alone in a ranch-type home. He is diagnosed with OA. He was referred to occupational therapy for energy conservation, work simplification, safety awareness, and adherence in relation to daily household tasks. He reports high levels of hip and knee pain if he has to stand, bend, or walk for longer than 5 minutes. He has no adaptive equipment in his home. He indicates that he would like to be able to prepare simple meals for himself, complete his own grocery shopping, maintain a clean home, do his own laundry, and participate in some of his favorite leisure activities: playing cards with friends, gardening, and watching sporting events in person or on television.

1. What types of daily activities are appropriate for occupational therapy to consider with this client?
2. If Mr. Jones returned to his home, would he be safe in performing self-care and household activities? How could this client perform errands and tasks outside the home?
3. How could Mr. Jones perform leisure activities given his reports of pain and low endurance?
4. What evaluations, based on those described in this chapter, might be both beneficial and appropriate for Mr. Jones in regard to his current status and needs?
5. What occupational therapy interventions would be appropriate to help Mr. Jones attain his goals for the performance of household tasks?

Neurological

Mrs. Smith sustained a CVA 1 month ago. Her dominant right arm and hand were affected by the CVA, and she currently has present but weak active motion in her dominant right arm. She plans on returning home to reside with her husband and adult child in their two-story home. The home is only accessible by five steps with a wrought-iron railing in the front and attached garage access followed by six steps up to the main living level at the side entrance of the home. She indicates that she was the primary house manager, taking care of cleaning, laundry, grocery shopping, bills, etc., whereas her husband took care of home maintenance, outside lawn and garden care, and any renovations of home maintenance issues. She states, "This is how it has always been." At this time, she is ambulating with a RLE brace and a cane, due to RLE instability and weakness. She is only able to walk for distances less than 50 feet before needing to stop and rest.

1. Based on this limited information, provide suggestions for adaptive equipment or DME that will help this client to be independent, or at least less dependent, upon her return home.
2. Can you suggest any home modifications that will enable Mrs. Smith to move about more freely in her home? If so, what are your suggestions?
3. Because Mrs. Smith wants to resume doing her daily occupations that she assumed before her CVA, what suggestions could you make to enable her to be more independent in her daily household tasks at this time?

Cardiac

Mr. Johnson sustained an MI approximately 1 week ago. He will be returning to his condo where he resides with his wife. He is depressed and reports that he feels he will die soon because of the MI. He indicates that he feels that his "life is over" because he will not be able to walk, golf, or engage in intimate sexual activity with his spouse. He does not readily engage in any occupational therapy interventions, such as dressing or grooming; he complains about "this horrible food—it's tasteless"; and he has adopted a rather gruff attitude toward family and friends who have come to visit him on the cardiac unit. He will be returning home tomorrow and reports that he is not looking forward to returning home to his wife and his familiar surroundings.

1. What types of in-clinic activities could be presented to this client to prepare him for his return home?
2. Because of Mr. Johnson's concerns about his intimate relationship with his wife, how could you broach the subject of sexuality with him?

SUMMARY

Because of the diversity of diagnoses and client characteristics in this practice setting, therapists must be familiar with the diagnosis, client characteristics, screens, evaluations, and interventions most appropriate for their client group. A solid general understanding of physical disabilities and the role of occupational therapist in the particular facility will help consolidate practice and enhance client progress. Physical disability practice is rewarding for the therapist and beneficial for the client.

QUESTIONS TO CONSIDER FOR STUDENT LEARNING AND REASONING

1. Identify why it is important for any student to have a broad understanding of a variety of physical disabilities.
2. If your client desires to return to his or her home, why is the performance of a home evaluation a necessity? Is a home evaluation necessary if the client is returning home and has either family or a designated caregiver?
3. Your client does not want to participate in your morning ADL bathing, grooming, dressing, and transferring session. The client reports that his significant other takes care of these things and he does not want to become involved in this process. Are ADL a major part of occupational therapy? Does every client need this type of training or retraining? If so, why; and if not, why not? What evaluation might provide you with additional information regarding this issue?

REFERENCES

Annon, J. (1976). The PLISSIT model: A proposed behavioral scheme for the behavioral treatment of sexual problems. *Journal of Sex Education Therapy*, 2(1), 1–15.

Baum, C., Monison, T., Hahn, M., & Edwards, D.F. (2003). *Test manual: Executive Function Performance Test*. St. Louis, MO: Washington University.

Calman, K.C. (1984). Quality of life in cancer patients: An hypothesis. *Journal of Medical Ethics*, 10, 3, 124-127.

Centers for Disease Control and Prevention. (2014c). *Traumatic brain injury*. Retrieved from http://www.cdc.gov/TraumaticBrainInjury/index.html

DeRosa, J. (2013, September 23). Providing self-management support to people living with chronic conditions. *OT Practice*, CE-1–CE-7.

Fisher, A. (1999). *Assessment of Motor and Process Skills* (3rd ed.). Ft. Collins, CO: Three Star Press.

Gould, B., & Dyer, R. (2011). *Pathophysiology for health professions* (4th ed.). St. Louis, MO: Saunders/Elsevier.

Hart, J., & Loeffler, A. (2012). The endocrine system. In J. Hart & A. Loeffler (Eds.), *An introduction to human disease: Pathophysiology for healthcare professionals*. (379) Sudbury, MA: Jones & Bartlett Learning.

Hattjar, B. (2012). *Sexuality and occupational therapy: Strategies for persons with disabilities*. Bethesda, MD: AOTA Press.

Healthy People 2020. (2010). Health-Related Quality of Life and Well-Being. Retrieved from http://www.cdc.gov/nchs/healthy_peoplehp2020.htm

Heinmann, N. E., Allen C. K., & Yerxa, E. J. (1989). The routine task inventory: A tool for describing the functional behaviors of the cognitively disabled. *OT Practice, 1*, 67–74.

Katz, A. (2007). Sexuality and myocardial infarction. *American Journal of Nursing, 107*(3), 49–52.

Kohlman Thompson, L. (2016). *Kohlman Evaluation of Living Skills (KELS)*, 4th ed., p1. Bethesda, MD: AOTA Press.

Kramer, J., Kielhofner, G., & Forsyth, K. (2012). Assessments using the model of human occupation. In: B. Hemphill-Pearson (Ed.), *Assessments in Occupational Therapy Mental Health: An Integrated Approach* (2nd ed., pp. 173–175). Thorofare, NJ: SLACK Incorporated.

Law, M., Baptiste, S., Carswell, A., McColl, M.A., Polatajko, H., & Pollock, N. (2005). *The Canadian Occupational Performance Measure*. Ottawa, CA: Canadian Association of Occupational Therapy.

Matthews, Brander. (1914). *The Oxford Book of American Essays*. New York, NY: Oxford University Press.

Mayo Clinic. (2014). *Diseases and conditions: Parkinson's disease*. Retrieved from http://www.mayoclinic.org/diseases-conditions/parkinsons-disease/basics/definition/con-20028488?p=1

McGourty, L. K. (1979). *Kohlman evaluation of living skills*. Seattle, WA: KELS Research.

Michael J. Fox Foundation. (2018). Our Role and Impact: Michael's Story. Retrieved from: http://www.michaeljfoxfoundation.org

Millard, D. R. (1986). Primary wound closure. In *Principalization of plastic surgery*. Boston, MA. Little, Brown.

National Multiple Sclerosis Society. (2018). *Definition of MS*. Retrieved from http://www.nationalmssociety.org/What-is-MS/Definition-of-MS

National Multiple Sclerosis Society. (n.d.-b). *Who gets MS (Epidemiology)*. Retrieved from: https://www.nationalmssociety.org/What-is-MS/Who-Gets-MS

PA Health Law Project. (2014). *Letter of medical necessity*. Retrieved from http://www.pahealthlaw-project.com

Sladyk, K., Jacobs, K., & MacRae, N. (2010). *Occupational therapy essentials for clinical competence*. Thorofare, NJ: SLACK Incorporated.

Practice in Pediatrics and Work With Individuals Under Age 18 Years

KEY WORDS

- Adaptive response
- Developmental vs chronological age
- Developmental milestones
- Play
- Sensory integration and sensory processing

Hattjar, B.
*Fundamentals of Occupational Therapy:
An Introduction to the Profession* (pp. 59-70).

Throughout the history of the occupational therapy profession, practitioners have focused on the evaluation and treatment of people who are experiencing the effects of illness, injury, or disability. In the pediatric setting, this initially took place in traditional hospitals where "sick" children were receiving medical care. The focus of occupational therapy was to provide the opportunity for and guidance in maintaining old skills and learning new ones, by assisting the children in making healthy adjustments and by discerning and meeting many of their normal needs. This type of intervention and care is representative of the medical model of care. With the doctor, nurse, and teacher, the occupational therapist contributes to an environment promoting the growth of the ill and handicapped child to a healthier adulthood.

As the scope of the profession grew and the health care environment changed, occupational therapists began to provide services to children, youth, and adolescents in schools, clients' home, outpatient settings, and traditional hospital settings. The focus of occupational therapy has shifted to supporting a students (or child's) ability participate in daily (school) activities "occupations" (American Occupational Therapy Association [AOTA], 2018). Occupational therapy helps to support daily childhood, youth, or adolescent occupations including that of a student, playmate, son or daughter, or friend by supporting achievement, active engagement, and learning. Whereas the therapist in the 20th century would intervene with ill and handicapped individuals, occupational therapists now provide services to an extremely wide variety of individuals under the age of 18 years of age in diverse settings.

The role of occupational therapy and pediatrics has expanded so much that this type of work comprises one of the largest employment areas for occupational therapy practitioners (AOTA, 2014).

SERVICE LOCATIONS

In the late 20th and early 21st centuries, occupational therapists have provided evaluation and treatment in the following settings to children, youth, and adolescents with relevant diagnosis:

- School-based services: Occupational therapists and occupational therapy assistants provide services that are determined to be "educationally relevant" and those that help children "to prepare for and perform important learning and school related activities and to fulfill their role as students" (AOTA, 2014). This includes working with children who have problems with skills that impede their ability to learn, function, and progress in academic areas including, but not limited to, writing, reading, functional mobility, socialization, and math skills.
- Inpatient services: Services provided by practitioners in the inpatient setting relate to medical diagnoses and the improved status of the child. Usually, once medical issues are resolved, the child is referred to a less intensive therapeutic or treatment environment, such as the home, outpatient, or pediatric rehabilitation, or for monitoring in the school-based setting. Children's length of stay in

an inpatient facility is determined by their diagnosis and the severity of their illness, injury, or disability.

- Outpatient services: Outpatient occupational therapy services can be varied and include, but are not limited to, services used to augment or supplement school-based services; motor deficits including balance deficits; *sensory integration* or *sensory processing* deficits; vision problems; memory problems; performance (of gross or fine motor) issues; strength, endurance, and range-of-motion problems; activities of daily living issues, including dressing, grooming, transferring, and bathing; and developmental issues. Outpatient treatment tends to address occupational deficits in typical childhood roles of student, sibling, family member, and social being.

- Community-based services: The type of community-based service the practitioner provides is dictated by the intent of the community-based facility. In the case of afterschool programming, the focus of therapy may be the completion of homework, computer use, socialization, motor problems, or health and wellness (e.g., obesity-focused programming). Additionally, community-based programming may focus on bullying, communication skills, or *play* skills depending on the focus of the facility and the needs of the children involved in programming. The focus in a community-based setting is reflective of the mission of the facility and the community as a whole.

- Clinic services: Clinics are designed to meet the needs of a specific deficit area, such as assistive technology or orthopedics. Therefore, therapeutic interventions provided by practitioners would focus solely on the intent of the service clinic. In the clinic setting, children and their families may travel long distances (e.g., when they reside in rural settings) to obtain services that might otherwise be unavailable to them.

- Home care services: These services, provided in the child's natural home environment, are designed to address specific deficits related to the child's diagnosis. Home-based services may be provided to children receiving early intervention programming (generally provided to children from birth through age 3 years) before they are old enough to qualify for or attend out-of-home services. Home care also addresses the needs of children who are very ill and cannot travel to other service settings. By working with a child in the most natural of settings—the home—the therapist can also assess the family and provide education.

PEDIATRIC DIAGNOSIS GROUPS

The following represents a few of the many diagnosis groups that pediatric occupational therapists work with to promote occupational well-being and life engagement:

- Autism spectrum disorders: This diagnosis category has been expanded in the fifth edition of the *Diagnostic and Statistical Manual of Mental Disorders* (DSM–5; American Psychiatric Association [APA], 2013). Whereas many of the diagnosis included in this spectrum used to be singled out or individualized in previous

DSM editions, the *DSM–5* seeks to place diagnoses such as Asperger's syndrome, autism, Rett's syndrome, and sensory processing disorders on a continuum of severity, rather than in separate and distinct categories or diagnosis areas (APA, 2013). These disorders all have specific symptoms, but the key is the level of severity or involvement the problems express in a particular child; although they share typical social, interactional, and intellectual issues, the level of severity and life involvement differs significantly. The placement of these disorders on the "autistic spectrum" is, at this time, controversial for some practitioners, educators, parents or caregivers, and insurance companies. However, the spectrum eliminates categorizing, labeling, and stigmatizing of the diagnosed child.

- Developmental disabilities/intellectual disabilities: Previously referred to as mental retardation, the descriptive names of these disorders, intellectual disability (ID) and developmental disability, reflect the essence of the diagnosis. IDs are intellectual limitations that affect learning, motor, and psychological development and maturation. The ability to perform typical daily tasks may be impeded, and the ability to communicate and live independently is usually affected in some way. Intelligence quotient (IQ) is one measure of ID. It is generally considered that an IQ of 70 or lower places an individual at the level of disability. The lower the IQ, therefore, the greater the effect of this disability. Frequently, ID is diagnosed before the child enters first grade. ID is a lifelong disability.

  Developmental disabilities have an impact on a child's normal progression through *developmental milestones* that include motor, psychological, and intellectual aspects. Developmental disability is a more general category than ID, and therefore, it can affect a number of typical life roles, such as being a student, son or daughter, sibling, or playmate.

- Cerebral palsy: This disorder is characterized by nonprogressive abnormal muscular coordination with or without ID or seizure disorders. It is sometimes caused by brain damage or injury that occurs in the late fetal or perinatal period of life. Cerebral palsy is a one-time insult to the brain that does not progress but frequently causes developmental, social, mobility, and possibly intellectual problems for the person. Although the physical problems associated with cerebral palsy can be significant, the intellectual and developmental issues may also present developmental limitations and deterrents.

- Prematurity: Prematurity is the most important cause of disease during the perinatal period. This refers to infants born at or before 37 weeks' gestation. Approximately 10% of all live births are premature. Premature babies run a higher risk of developing pneumonia or hyaline membrane disease (which affects the infant's immature lungs), neurologic damage resulting from intracranial hemorrhages, severe intestinal tract infections, sepsis, and severe retinal damage (Loeffler & Hart, 2015). The effects of any of these, or any combination of them, can result in significant impairment. Prematurity also correlates with low birth weight, another predisposing factor for infants.

In health care, the extent of an infant's prematurity can be subtracted from his or her *chronological age* (Box 4-1); this number represents the actual chronological and *developmental age*. If a child is 6 months old chronologically but was born 6 weeks

Box 4-1
CALCULATING CHRONOLOGICAL AGE

Where the developmental age of a child is usually calculated through evaluation and assessment, the chronological (or birth age) of a child can be calculated as follows:

Current Year	Current Month	Current Day	2015	01	02
Birth Year	Birth Month	Birth Day	2005	11	05

Consider that a year has 12 months, and generalize to assume that each month has 30 days. Work from right to left and "borrow" as necessary:

You would "borrow" from the month column = 30 days for 1 month

You would "borrow" from the year column = 12 months for 1 year

The final answer to the problem above is 9 years, 1 month, 27 days

Another example:

2015	12	15	
2000	10	10 =	15 years, 2 months, 5 days

prematurely, the child should be expected to be performing developmental tasks similar to a 4.5-month-old baby. With the support of therapy, this difference can be minimized and eliminated over time. However, the greater the difference between chronological and developmental age, the greater the disability.

- Chromosomal diseases: Some examples of chromosomal diseases include Down syndrome, Klinefelter syndrome, Fragile X syndrome, and Turner syndrome. Of these diagnoses, probably the most well know is Down syndrome or trisomy 21. In the past, this syndrome was referred to as *mongolism* because people with Down syndrome characteristically possess slanted eyes due to an extra ocular skinfold. This term is no longer commonly used or considered appropriate. Along with the particular presentation of the eyes, these individuals tend to have lower than average IQ; an additional fold in their palms called a *simian crease;* a rather "chubby" looking or protruding abdomen (due to low muscle tone and strength); and problems with vision, speech, and gross and fine motor skills. As children, they tend to reach developmental milestones at a later age and may "peak" in developmental progression at a young age. They tend to be pleasant in nature, exhibit low muscle tone, walk with a wide-based or shuffling gait pattern, have vision and cataract problems, and speak in a voice that is considered to be more nasal in tone.

In the past, people with Down syndrome tended not to live past their third decade. Due to medical advancements, they are living longer—into their 40s, 50s or 60s—and are experiencing the effects of aging, like arthritis and DAT, earlier than the normal population. Rapid aging symptoms include skin wrinkling; lack of skin elasticity; vision and age-related vision problems like cataracts, macular degeneration, and presbyopia; arthritis in weightbearing joints and osteoarthritis; and early menopause for women, among other age-related symptoms that appear earlier than people who do not have Down syndrome. However, current research also indicates that they are predisposed to early-onset dementia of the Alzheimer's type (or dementia that closely resembles Alzheimer's disease) by the late third or fourth decade of life (Alzheimer's Association, n.d.; Cleveland Clinic, 2011).

- Fragile X syndrome: This is characterized by mild to moderate ID and it is the most common cause of ID in males. Individuals afflicted with Fragile X syndrome have a characteristic long face and enlarged ears (Loeffler & Hart, 2015), and the extent of the ID varies.

- Klinefelter syndrome: This syndrome affects boys and men who have one Y and two X chromosomes, which represents a sex chromosome trisomy. This syndrome is usually not diagnosed until right before or during puberty. It presents with symptoms such as male breast enlargement and the lack of the development of secondary male sex characteristics. People with Klinefelter usually respond well to testosterone therapy but are at risk for the development of breast cancer. The inclusion of testosterone therapy usually allows men with the syndrome to father children. As younger children, clients with Klinefelter syndrome also tend to experience language difficulties or delays (Loeffler & Hart, 2015).

- Turner syndrome: Clients with this diagnoses are female. Rather than a trisomy characteristic, this is a sex characteristic monosomy. People with this syndrome fail to go through female secondary sex characteristic development, are short in stature, and have a broad neck. They do not experience ID, however (Loeffler & Hart, 2015).

SENSORY INTEGRATION AND SENSORY PROCESSING DISORDERS

Sensory integration disorder (or dysfunction) is a neurological disorder that results from the brain's inability to integrate certain information received from the body's five major senses (thefreedictionary.com, 2015), as well as tactile (touch), proprioceptive (sense of self/position of the self), and vestibular (balance/head position sense) systems (as identified by A. Jean Ayres; Cole, 2012). These sensory systems are responsible for detecting sight, sound, smell, taste, temperature, pain, head position, and the body position and movement. The brain forms a combined picture of the information it receives to make sense of and react appropriately to the input (the appropriate *adaptive response*). The Sensory Integration theory was first put forth by A. Jean Ayres, PhD, OTR, in the 1980s, although her research on sensory integration began in the 1960s with children diagnosed as having "learning disabilities." It is interesting to note that Dr. Ayres' interest in this topic first began when she worked with children who were diagnosed with cerebral palsy.

Sensory integration is automatic for most people. For those with a sensory integration problem, this process is inefficient or incorrect, and the integration component is not present. The sensory integration process begins at birth and continues throughout life, although the majority of sensory integration occurs during childhood. The ability for sensory integration to become more accurate, refined, and effective coincides with the aging or maturation process in regard to motor, speech, and emotional-psychological development (thefreedictionary.com, 2015).

Although similar to sensory integration, sensory processing deals with how an individual responds and reacts to sensory input that supports or interferes with functional performance (Dunn, 2008). This deals with preferences (e.g., staying indoors rather than going outdoors; wearing shoes as opposed to going barefoot; preferring certain types of clothing; preferring certain types of food; experiencing adverse and out-of-proportion reactions to textures, closeness of others, touch, sound interpretation and level) and aversions to situations, people, and external and internal sensations. Sensory processing deficiencies are well assessed by the Sensory Profile (Dunn, 2008).

It is important to note that the diagnoses described here represent only a small number of those with which pediatric occupational therapists commonly work.

WORK AS AN OCCUPATIONAL THERAPIST IN THE PEDIATRIC ARENA

The pediatric occupational therapist must possess a wide variety of skills and be creative, patient, and positive and welcoming to children. Many times, children will fail to "separate" easily from the parent or caregiver when treatment is about to begin, and this is frequently due to behavioral issues, anxiety about exactly what therapy will consist of, and because of past "scary" experiences with members of the health care professions (e.g., when getting vaccinations, blood tests, x-rays). Sometimes, it is prudent to have the parent or caregiver observe the first therapy or evaluation session because this usually decreases a child's anxiety and fear. This tends to work well in inpatient and outpatient settings. In school settings, the therapist must be warm, positive, and welcoming to the child as a session begins.

It is also important to engage child clients in conversation, let them make some activity or therapy toy selections, and have them be comfortably involved with the therapy process. However, it is also important to have clear rules or norms for therapy, such as following your directions, listening to your words, and staying on task for the duration of the activity as much as possible. When working with children, a reward system for staying on task may be used to encourage positivity and good work in therapy. Remember that this is therapy, not just play—although good therapy tends to look like play! This dichotomy presents a significant learning curve for most therapists but is accomplished with experience and supervision from an experienced practitioner or mentor or through involvement in continuing education programs.

The pediatric occupational therapist must exhibit a desire to work with children and be adept in handling their needs, both physical and emotional. The therapist must have a good energy level, be creative, and also be physically able to assume a variety of positions (for demonstration and play-based tasks) and execute movements such as jumping, hopping, and skipping. Because working with children can sometimes be emotionally challenging (consider crying or inconsolable children, oppositional children, or those who refuse to cooperate and thereby endanger their—and your—safety in the therapy session), the therapist must have a strong constitution and sense of self as a competent practitioner. The therapist must be able to focus solely on the child and ensure safety in therapy. Remember that parents, teachers, and caregivers are entrusting their child to your care, and this is a great responsibility.

The general work skills necessary for pediatric therapists include knowledge of normal versus abnormal development and of reflex persistence and integration (Fiorentino, 1978) as well as the ability to clearly explain anything to a child in language that they will understand. Therapists must also be able to gain both the child's and the parent's, teacher's, or caregiver's trust and respect within the therapy arena. Because home, classroom, or outside of therapy carryover is important, this is a crucial element for the pediatric therapist as well. This does involve getting the child and caregiver to carryover therapy items to the out of therapy environments. This can be accomplished by the child practicing skills in therapy, the caregiver observing therapy and trying skill sets in therapy with the child, and by providing handouts or brochures detailing techniques or activities that should be conducted outside of therapy to support therapy interventions.

WHAT DOES PEDIATRIC OCCUPATIONAL THERAPY LOOK LIKE? IS IT PLAY OR NOT?

Play is usually considered a major childhood occupation and role (having or being a playmate), although as we mature, the word *play* becomes replaced with words such as *hobbies*, *leisure*, or *recreation* (Kuhaneck, Spitzer, & Miller, 2010). Play should be considered the major activity that prepares children for ongoing development in motor, social, and cognitive areas. Play skills can be generalized into "working" or playing with other people; gaining an understanding of teamwork; doing something that is motivating, fun, and interesting; and doing something that calms, organizes, or reduces anxiety or fear. Not all play is "just fun," and play can have fear or anxiety components associated with its execution, but the connecting element is that play involves many types of learning depending on the particular play activity as well as the needs of the child (Box 4-2).

Children understand play, and its components are important for therapy sessions. The therapy environment should be welcoming and warm and have an adequate supply of equipment, toys, and other objects to make it an atmosphere with which children want to interact. Therapy clinics or rooms frequently have a large, open space for gross motor tasks, and pediatric-sized tables and chairs for fine motor activities, testing, crafts, and tabletop game tasks. Storage is also an important clinic element because items should be stored and then brought out for therapy sessions. If a child is easily distractible or has a short attention span, easy access to objects such as balls

Box 4-2
COMMON CHARACTERISTICS OF ACTIVITIES DEFINED AS PLAY
Flexibility
Spontaneity
Intrinsic motivation
Nonliteral or symbolic use of objects
Voluntary engagement
Free choice
Elicitation of positive affect (fun/enjoyable)
Lack of functional or purposeful goals
Often resembles real behaviors but lacks the consequences of real behaviors
Kuhaneck, Spitzer & Miller, 2010

and scooter boards can prove to be a safety and focus issue in therapy. The pediatric clinic usually has climbing, swinging, and positioning equipment as well.

Most therapy areas have and use tools that "look like" play items or toys but have a therapeutic benefit when used with a child. A large therapy ball can be used to learn ball skills but also to strengthen weak muscles, promote balance, and challenge endurance and strength. Scooter boards can be used for "just-fun" speed racing but are also used to promote stability, balance, prone positioning, speed tolerance, and both upper and lower extremity strength and agility related to prone and sometimes supine positioning. Computers can be used for computer games but also to improve visual motor skills, finer isolation through keying, right and left discrimination, focus and attention, color identification, reading skill improvement, and eye-tracking skills. Swinging items such as bolsters or net swings can be used for swinging and movement integration but can also be used for trunk stabilization and vestibular integration. Therefore, therapy should "look like" play but have additional therapeutic purpose. If the therapist is only using the tools for "fun," it is not therapy; it is play. Play is an essential component of any therapy session, but it should always be used for therapeutic means. How this is accomplished depends on the creativity, comfort, and knowledge of the occupational therapist.

PEDIATRIC EVALUATIONS

A wide variety of therapeutic evaluations exist. The types of evaluations used by the therapist are dictated by the child's age, diagnosis, and needs. The following represent some of the commonly used pediatric evaluations occupational therapists use:

- Batelle Developmental Inventory: This test evaluates early childhood developmental milestones. The Batelle test is designed for children from birth through age 8 years. It tests several developmental domains, including self-help, motor (both gross and fine), cognition, language, and social skills (Houghton Mifflin Harcourt, 2018). Administration of the Batelle takes about 1 hour. There is a short screening version that takes about 30 minutes for administration. This test is a "child-friendly" assessment because it uses play-based items that appeal to children.

- Brunincks Oseretsky Test-II (BOT-II): The BOT-II is an individually administered test that uses engaging, goal-directed activities to measure a wide array of motor skills in children, adolescents, and young adults aged 4 through 21 years (Lynne Oberle, EdD, OTR, verbal communication, 2015). The BOT-II is one of the few evaluations that covers this wide age span. It includes a full version that takes about 1 hour and a short version that takes about 20 to 30 minutes to complete. This test has been in use for many years and continues to be a frequent choice among occupational therapists.

- Developmental Test of Visual Perception, 2nd edition (DVPT-II): The DVPT-II consists of eight subtests grouped into two categories: visual perception and visual-motor integration (Lynne Oberle, EdD, verbal interview, 2015). This test discriminates visual problems that can impede a child's academic and social development and interfere with psychological maturation.

- Evaluation Tool of Children's Handwriting (ETCH): The ETCH measures a child's handwriting speed and legibility skills in Grades 1 through 6 for the following: manuscript/printing and cursive/handwriting. [Domains (manuscript/print or cursive/writing)]. Included in this test are alphabet writing of lowercase and uppercase letters, numeral writing, near-point copying, far-point copying, manuscript/print to cursive/writing transition, dictation (writing or printing stated words), and sentence composition (Eastern Kentucky University Handwriting Assessment Tools, 2015).

- Sensory Integration and Praxis Test (SIPT): Considered by many professionals to be the gold standard for the testing of sensory integration problems, the SIPT requires extensive training and is only administered by practitioners who are certified to do so. The training process for therapists is both extensive and expensive. The SIPT assesses a wide composite of sensory integration components and comes with an extensive test kit. This test is time-consuming, and test results must be calculated through a computer program for scoring purposes. It must also be explained to parents or caregivers in lay terms to ensure their understanding of the results. Children tend to find this test interesting and engaging. The SIPT is a revision of A. Jean Ayres' Southern California Sensory Integration Test; as noted earlier, Ayres is credited with the development of sensory integration theory and treatment and intervention approaches for sensory issues. Dr. Ayres defined sensory integrations as, "The neurological process that organizes sensation from one's own body and from the environment and makes it possible to use the body effectively within the environment" (Sensory Integration Network Ltd., 2018).

- Sensory Profile: This component of evaluation can be given to the parent or caregiver (infant or child editions); teachers, parents, or caregivers (school edition);

or the person being tested (adolescent/adult edition). The Sensory Profile can be administered in conjunction with the occupational therapy evaluation or as an adjunct to therapy. It is a report format, is easy to score, and can substantiate evaluation findings related to sensory processing issues (Brown & Dunn, 2002; Dunn, 2008).

- Miller Assessment for Preschoolers (MAP): The MAP, developed by Lucy Miller, OTR, is a relatively short but comprehensive preschool evaluation that assesses mild to moderate developmental delays. Test items in the MAP are objective, and the test is easy to administer. The MAP provides the practitioner with a broad overview of a child's developmental status compared with other children of the same age (Banus, 1983). The test is appealing and engaging for children due to the test activities and items included in the test kit.

- Peabody Developmental Motor Scales: The Peabody is a widely used assessment. It looks at a child's developmental status in children from birth through 7 years of age. The test measures gross and fine motor developmental skills through the use of typical motor activities (Markursic, 2012). In the author's opinion, this test does require the administrator to clearly understand the difference between normal and abnormal development in the birth through 7 years of age range.

SUMMARY

As occupational therapy has become a more recognized and better understood profession, the treatment of children with a wide variety of concerns has likewise increased. It is reasonable to assume that problems addressed earlier in life tend to be more "fixable" and more easily accommodated by diagnosed individuals and their significant others. Because of the plasticity of the nervous system and the overall maturation and developmental processes that occur in children, pediatric occupational therapy is beneficial and can produce lifelong benefits.

QUESTIONS TO CONSIDER FOR STUDENT LEARNING AND REASONING

1. How would you explain occupational therapy to a child's parents?
2. How would you explain occupational therapy to a 5-year-old? A 15-year-old?
3. Your child client refuses to complete a therapy task with you and asks to do something else. How would you deal with this situation? Can you set norms or limits with a child?
4. After completing an assessment with a child, you always review the results with the parents or caregivers. The child has not done well on the evaluation, so how

do you temper your explanation to make it objective and positive, rather than subjective and negative?

5. Talking about therapy, your 13-year-old client states, "This is stupid and a waste of time." How would you explain the benefits of therapy to this young person in terms he or she would understand?

6. Identify three reinforcements to promote engagement in therapy for a 5-year-old and for a 15-year-old.

REFERENCES

Alzheimer's Association. (n.d.). *Down syndrome and Alzheimer's disease.* Retrieved from http://alz.org/dementia/down-syndrome-alzheimers-symptoms.asp

American Occupational Therapy Association. (2018). *School-based occupational therapy fact sheet.* Retrieved from: https://www.aota.org/About-Occupational-Therapy/Professionals/CY/School.aspx

American Occupational Therapy Association. (2014). *Occupational therapy in school settings.* Retrieved from https://www.aota.org/About-Occupational-Therapy/Professionals/CY/school-settings.aspx

American Psychiatric Association. (2013). *The diagnostic and statistical manual of mental disorders* (5th ed.). Washington, DC: Author.

Banus, B. (1983). The miller's assessment for preschoolers: An introduction and review. *American Journal of Occupational Therapy*, 37, 333-340.

Brown, C., & Dunn, W., (2002). *The adolescent and adult sensory profile.* New York, NY: Pearson Education.

Cleveland Clinic. (2011). *Alzheimer's disease and Down syndrome.* Retrieved from https://my.clevelandclinic.org/health/diseases/9173-alzheimers-disease-and-down-syndrome

Cole, M. (2012). *Group dynamics in occupational therapy: The theoretical and practice application of group intervention.* Thorofare, NJ: SLACK Incorporated.

Dunn, W. (2008). *The sensory profile.* New York, NY: Pearson Education.

Eastern Kentucky University Handwriting Assessments. (2015). The ETCH. Retrieved from http://www.eku.edu/etch

Fiorentino, M. (1980). *The influence of primitive reflexes on motor development* (4th ed.). Springfield, IL: Charles C. Thomas.

Houghton Mifflin Harcourt. (2018). Batelle Developmental Inventory. Retrieved from: https://www.hmhco.com/programs/battelle-developmental-inventory

Kuhaneck, H., Spitzer, S. & Miller, E. (2010). *Activity analysis, creativity, and playfulness in pediatric occupational therapy: Making play just right.* Sudbury, MA: Jones & Bartlett Learning.

Loeffler, A., & Hart, M. (2015). *Introduction to human diseases: Pathophysiology for healthcare professionals* (6th ed.). Burlington, MA: Jones & Bartlett Learning.

Markursic, M. (2012). Peabody Developmental Motor Scales. Retrieved from: https://www.brighthubeducation.com/special-ed-physical-disabilities/13499-assess-the-motor-skills-of-children-using-peabody-developmental-motor-scale/

Miller, L., (2015). The Miller Assessment of Preschoolers. Retrieved from: http://Pearsonclinical.com./map

Sensory Integration Network, Ltd. (2018). Sensory integration education: What is sensory integration?, SI theory. Retrieved from: https://www.sensoryintegration.org.uk/

Theoretical Foundation, Frames of Reference, and Practice Models for the Occupational Therapy Profession

---

KEY WORDS

- Adaptive response
- Approach
- Frame of reference (FOR)
- Model
- Theory

Hattjar, B.
*Fundamentals of Occupational Therapy:
An Introduction to the Profession* (pp. 71-92).
© 2019 Taylor & Francis Group.

Theory provides a profession with a way to think about or perform an action. Theory provides occupational therapy with a structure and the resulting topics related to what we need to do and how we need to align our thinking when dealing with clients. It provides us with a way "to explain the relationship between people, health, environment and other factors" (Cole, 2012, p. 125); theory makes it "possible for [occupational therapists] to understand the complexity of occupation and the optimal participation in daily life" (Dunbar, 2007, p. 2, as cited in Cole, 2012, p. 125).

Some theories provide very structured methods and rationale, whereas other theoretical bases are somewhat vague or open-ended in their presentation. Some theoretical bases can be used alone, whereas other theoretical bases can be used in conjunction with other theoretical approaches. Some theoretical bases are better used with people who have psychological or psychiatric problems, some are better if used with those who have developmental issues, and some are better to use with those who have physical problems. It is up to the therapist both to understand and to implement the use of the most appropriate theories or theory when working with any client.

Theory can be confusing and difficult to grasp and use, or it can be a rather fascinating way to align evaluation, treatment, goals, and client progression within a treatment or clinical setting. I believe that theory can be interesting and enlightening in relation to selecting the best theoretical base and systematically selecting evaluations, developing goals, and providing interventions that meet the specification of the theory.

To understand the words—*theory, frame of reference* (FOR), *model*, and *approach*—frequently used interchangeably to describe what theory consider the following definitions:

- Theory: Theory is "a supposition or system of ideas intended to explain something, especially one based on general principles of (the) things to be explained" (Oxford Dictionary, 2018). Theory tells us the "why," "what," "how," and "when" about an action based on rules, ideas, etc. that are set forth within the theory. Theory does not always translate well into actual evaluation and practice, however. Those used in occupational therapy may originate from within or outside of the profession as well.
- FOR: A frame of reference is, "a set of beliefs or ideas on which you base your judgment of things" (Collins Dictionary, 2018). FORs address specific disabilities that create problems in occupational performance. They may draw on knowledge from both inside and outside of the profession The overarching goal of any FOR used in occupational therapy is to support client independence and engagement in meaningful and purposeful occupation.
- Model: Here *model* is used as in *model of practice*, that is, a compilation of "professional values, implementation, evaluation; the structure, process, and values that support care and the environment in which it is delivered" (Hoffart & Woods, 1996). A model identifies how something, such as a system, should work in occupational therapy, but it does not provide an actual direction for occupational therapy practice (Reed & Sanderson, 1999).

- Approach: This indicates a way of dealing with something; a way of doing or thinking about something (Merriam-Webster's Dictionary, 2018); in this context, consider an approach to be a distinct way of looking at and implementing components of a larger "whole" or a way of thinking and doing.

These terms can be confusing to both novice students and seasoned practitioners. It is important to realize that our professional, therapeutic actions have to be grounded in structure, and a theoretical framework FOR, model, or approach provides us with such a structure or system. Also, for the novice student, all of the particulars about the various theories can be overwhelming and not make sense at the entry level of gaining your professional knowledge. Therefore, the generalities in this chapter are provided to promote thinking and further investigation and knowledge acquisition, as opposed to detailing minutia. This will provide you with a basic idea about the wide variety of theories that influence and direct the profession of occupational therapy. This variety interfaces well with the occupational therapy profession because of the broadness and scope of the profession.

THEORIES FROM WITHIN OCCUPATIONAL THERAPY

To provide a more general view of theory, the first section of this chapter focuses exclusively on theories that have been developed within the profession and by occupational therapists.

Sensorimotor Theories and Sensory Integration

Theory Development

Sensorimotor approaches look at a variety of areas including, but not limited to, sensory, motor, perceptual, and cognitive developmental or acquired problems that affect the brain. Older sensorimotor approaches look at the developmental sequence and draw information from neurology and the neuroscience areas. More current sensorimotor theorists tend to look to a more client-centered approach (considering what a specific client needs) and focus on holism (treating the entire person to support engagement in occupational performance that is satisfying and appropriate for the individual) for evaluation and interventions.

Sensory Integration

The creation of the sensory integration model is attributed to Dr. Jean Ayres. Ayres' model was initially based on children who were diagnosed with cerebral palsy, then expanded to her observations of children diagnosed with learning disabilities (at the time of her observations, the terminology used was *minimal brain dysfunction* or *minimal brain damage*, terms that are now considered to be inaccurate and inappropriate). In her background research and observations, she noted neurological problems based on the inability to correctly process sensory information and make appropriate motor responses. This inability to correctly respond caused the children to react and respond in ways that were not developmentally appropriate or physically or psychologically aligned to the particular task demand. She indicated that an *adaptive response*—a response that met the task requirement(s) and was appropriate and adequate to the particular task—did not occur at all or did not occur with any regularity. In 1972, Ayres defined *sensory integration* as "the neurological process that organizes sensations from one's own body and from the environment and makes it possible to use the body effectively within the environment" (Sensory Integration Global Network, 2018). In her clinical observations, Ayres noted that children diagnosed with sensory integration problems did not automatically react or respond to sensory input, and this resulted in faulty sensory processing and output. Examples of this include distractibility when asked to focus on tasks, clumsiness or awkwardness when performing gross motor activities, difficulty easily transitioning from one activity to another, performance hesitation or fear and anxiety when asked to perform a motor activity, refusal to perform activities, decreased gross and fine motor skills that fell below age expectations for performance (e.g., writing, copying shapes, coloring, inconsistent or diminished grip patterns), behavioral problems, emotional lability, and, in more complex situations, social restriction, regression, and aggression. These children's performance created a multitude of occupational performance problems in school, at home, and in leisure and play activities. In current thinking, Ayres' sensory integration theory paved the way for what is now referred to as *sensory processing deficiencies*—that is, difficulty making appropriate and adaptive responses to incoming sensory input.

Sensory Integration Theory Concepts

- Neural plasticity is the brain's ability to be modified by ongoing input of sensory information, referred to as *sensory processing*. Additionally, this is integrated into evaluation and treatment through the use of developmentally appropriate and typical or normal activities or tasks. In other words, the more frequently a child has to make appropriate responses to an activity or task, the better he or she will be able to respond appropriately to sensory information through experience, learning, and performance (Kielhofner, 2009).

- According to this theory, sensory integration develops in a normal developmental progression; therefore, interventions using this model should follow the correct developmental sequence. This mandates that the child's correct chronological and developmental age be calculated at the time of evaluation or initial assessment (see Box 4-1 on how to calculate correct chronological age). Note that developmental age may be based on testing results provided in the evaluation of the child.

- The brain functions as an integrated whole. This means that if components of the whole are out of sync, this will affect the brain as a whole.

- Brain organization affects one's ability to make appropriate adaptive responses, and adaptive responses help to organize the brain. The process works in concert to promote effective and efficient integration of sensory information—that is, sensory processing.

- People have an innate drive to perform sensory-motor activities. Consider the play of a child—riding bicycles, running, skipping, jumping, jumping rope, dancing, playing sports and games; all require processing.

Evaluations Associated With Sensory Integration

The major evaluation used in the sensory integration model is the Sensory Integration and Praxis Test. To administer this evaluation, the occupational therapist must receive extensive training to correctly capture and execute this test and its subtests.

The Sensory Profile (Brown & Dunn, 2002) is also an evaluation component used with sensory integration and sensory processing problems. The Infant and Toddler and School-Based versions of this assessment component include a series of questions that are answered by the parent, caregiver, or, in the case of the school-based version, a teacher or an aide. An adolescent and adult version (Brown & Dunn, 2002) is also available. Therefore, the Sensory Profile can be used to augment information secured in an evaluation, and the profile is commonly used across the life span.

What Constitutes Sensory Integration Intervention?

Sensory integration interventions frequently look like play activities. As Piaget stated in regard to childhood play, "Play is the work of childhood", "Play is the answer to the question, and "How does anything new come about?" (Brainy Quotes, 2018). Through specific activities guided by client needs, the occupational therapist carefully and thoughtfully designs therapeutic activities that will engage the participant and promote an adaptive response—that is, an automatic, purposeful task-appropriate response to sensory stimuli (an activity component). For example, for an adult or child who has difficulty transitioning from one activity to another, has poor motor skills, and is fearful of movement, an obstacle course where the person is prone on a scooter board and must meet the task requirement of, for example, knocking down a cardboard "brick wall," move through a "dangerous route" where "alligators are close," and throwing a small therapy ball toward a desired target would meet a number of therapeutic needs, yet be a great fit for overall engagement and involvement. For a child who is somewhat defensive, perhaps a "find five jacks in a bowl of rice" might be a good activity, followed by placing the jacks in play dough or putty to hide them again. You could also have the child make the play dough to increase the amount of tactile input and to demonstrate the concept of following direction via the dough recipe. The possibilities are only limited by the occupational therapist's creativity and expertise in treatment. Additionally, either of these activities could promote learning engagement. People who have a positive experience in therapy tend to be more amenable to gym or recess activities. For clients who have issues with touch, therapy activities may help them be more assertive in their ability and desire to touch and do hand activities.

The *Model of Human Occupation* (MOHO) is attributed to Dr. Gary Kielhofner. The MOHO is accepted worldwide and is a broad approach to guiding and directing clients to look at and experience their needs and their responses to environmental input. The major focus of this theory is to improve an individual's participation and

---

Box 5-1

THE BASIC MOHO FEEDBACK LOOP

The MOHO Feedback Loop includes the following:

1. The process is initiated by input to the person from the environment.
2. The person processes this information based on one's habits and routines (habituation), activity motivation and choice (volition), and thoughts and feelings about his or her personal capacities and effectiveness (personal causation; relates to and is influenced by an individual's values and interests).
3. This is followed by the individual's output based on his or her processing.
4. The output to the environment secures feedback, which influences the next "dose" of input, and the feedback loop continues in this dynamic manner.

---

adaptation in life occupations (Kielhofner, 2009, p. 149). Client responses to input are reflected in their processing, consisting of habituation, volition, and personal causation. These three aspects comprise and contribute to the client response, or output. This feedback is interpreted, and input, throughput, and output continue in an evolving and ongoing process. The MOHO is a dynamic, fluid theory. It can be used with almost any client across the life span and with other theories or alone in some cases.

Kielhofner indicated that the powerful influence of occupation directs a person through his or her life. This includes the person's internal and external experiences; engagement in occupation is the result of the environment and the person's characteristics, and the internal characteristics (which may also be thought of as responses that are influenced by experience and personality) of an individual can be changed through occupational engagement. A good way to understand the MOHO is to look at the MOHO Feedback Loop (Box 5-1).

Kielhofner and Burke (1980, as cited in Kielhofner, 2009) stated that the MOHO is applicable for use with clients who are experiencing problems with:

- The motivation for occupation
- Maintaining positive involvement in life roles and routines
- Skilled performance of necessary life tasks
- The influence of the physical and social environment

To gain a visual picture of this theory, consider the outline of a large circle. Input is the information emanating from the outside; move forward on the circle outline to "throughput" consisting of habits, volition, and personal causation. These three factors promote our response based on the nature of the input and the manner in which we process the input. How we process this as an individual prompts our response(s) or our output to the outside. How we respond contributes to the feedback we receive. This feedback provides our input. This dynamic "circle" of feedback and response affects the dynamic, ever-changing feedback loop associated with the MOHO.

Because of the individual and personal mechanisms that figure prominently in this theory, it can be used with a wide variety of diagnosis groups, ages, and cultures.

How Would Therapy Work Using the MOHO?

Using the MOHO as the primary theoretical approach to therapy promotes a multitude of options for the therapist. This theory is applicable to a client base as diverse as working with a parent who is underemployed but who wishes to improve the job interviewing skills to secure a better form of employment, with a breast cancer survivor to promote a better and accurate body image, to the caregiver of a loved one with Alzheimer's disease who needs to relearn how to take care of herself first via better use of leisure time and hobbies. Therapeutic interventions can include physical, cognitive and behavioral, play-related, creative, and interactional/social and educational activities. The diversity of this theory also makes the MOHO an excellent choice to use in conjunction with other theoretical approaches such as those reviewed in this chapter. The MOHO has many screens and assessments associated with it and these can be accessed online for ordering purposes (search "The MOHO Web"). The MOHO is a dynamic and diverse theory that is well respected and frequently used in the profession of occupational therapy.

The intentional relationship (IR) model is attributed to Dr. Renee Taylor (2008) and constitutes an updated and revised consolidation of what used to be termed *therapeutic use of self* (Frank, 1958). This model describes the structure, process, and values that direct care. In general terms, occupational therapists have always been aware of how the personality dynamics between a client and therapist affect and flavor the therapeutic relationship. The major thrust of therapy was and is to engage and promote occupational involvement on the part of the client. As Taylor noted, "the therapist's role previously was to appropriately orient the client to occupations that were used as therapy"; however, according to IR theory, "the relationship between the therapist and the client [is] the key dynamic in therapy" (Taylor, 2008, p. 7). Ten underlying principles guide this theoretical model and approach:

1. Critical self-awareness is key to the intentional use of self; in other words, "therapist, know thyself!"
2. Interpersonal self-discipline is fundamental to the effective use of self; be aware of your own level of skill and knowledge and recognize biases and prejudices.
3. It is necessary to follow your head before your heart; be objective and empathetic.
4. Mindful empathy is required to know your client; sympathy and personal reactions do not correspond to your role as a professional therapist.
5. Therapists are responsible for expanding their personal knowledge base; stay current and maintain clear awareness of professional updates, changes, and knowledge.
6. Provided that they are purely and flexibly applied, a wide range of therapeutic modes can work and be used interchangeably in occupational therapy; retain creativity, theory knowledge, and concepts of "how and what" from various theoretical approaches that can be used to benefit the client.
7. The client defines a successful relationship.
8. Activity focusing must be balanced with interpersonal focusing.

9. Application of the model must be informed by core values and ethics of the profession.

10. Application of the model requires cultural competence, along with societal understanding of current trends and concerns (Taylor, 2008).

To use IR theory, the therapist must have active listening skills; possess good verbal communication (at a level of the client's understanding, and not "talking at" the client but "talking with" the client); be aware of nonverbal mannerisms and communication idioms; ask for and respond to client feedback; and provide structure, direction, and feedback to facilitate occupational engagement and involvement.

The IR model works in parallel with other theories and should be thought of as a necessary part of all therapeutic relationships. According to this theory, if a therapist does not know who he or she is as a person and does not adhere to high personal and professional standards and guidelines, therapy will not be therapeutic and may be riddled with personal biases, which may not prove to be beneficial to clients.

Allen's Cognitive Approach

Claudia Allen's theory has been evolving since the 1970s and is based on the premise that functional behavior is based on cognition. To produce more functional behavior, the thinking process must change (Cole, 2012). Allen's approach is strongly aligned with occupational therapy precepts because a client's performance in a task is determined by his or her ability to problem solve and be safe when doing a task. With many disabilities, these issues become impaired or disappear.

Claudia Allen is probably known best for her Allen Cognitive Level Screen (ACLS), a relatively quick and easy-to-administer leather-lacing screen. The leather stitches used in this screen are, first, a simple "running" of basting stitch, then a more complex whip stitch, followed by the third and last stitch, a more complicated single cordovan stitch. This screen provides us with an estimate of the client's best ability to function based on observation of a clients' activity or task performance (Allen, 1995). Allen has developed many other assessments, including the Routine Task Inventory and the Cognitive Performance Test. Where the ACLS uses leather lacing to determine cognitive levels, the Routine Task Inventory and Cognitive Performance Test use everyday activities and observation. Allen's most recent assessment, the Allen Diagnostic Module, uses standardized, prepackaged craft activities to determine cognitive levels and also takes into account the effect of socialization and motivation in this situation (Cole, 2012).

Through the "doing" process included in Allen's screens and assessments, we are able to observe, and then determine the client's cognitive levels (Box 5-2).

Allen has also broken down the six levels into modes of performance. The modes are percentile "pieces" of each level and provide even more information about the client's cognition and safety in task performance. They are identified as, for example, 3.8. This means the client is functioning at level 3; the .8 represents higher level 3 function (Box 5-3) as determined by the mode progression.

Box 5-2				

TITLES OF THE COGNITIVE LEVELS AND MODES OF PERFORMANCE FOR ALLEN COGNITIVE SCALES'S HIERARCHY OF FUNCTIONAL COGNITION

TITLE OF COGNITIVE LEVELS	TITLE OF MODES OF PERFORMANCE				
	.0	.2	.4	.6	.8
	Coma				0.8 Generalized reflexive actions
Level 1: Automatic Actions	1.0 Withdrawing from noxious stimuli	1.2 Responding to stimuli in 1 sensory system	1.4 Locating stimuli	1.6 Rolling body in bed	1.8 Raising body part
Level 2: Postural Actions	2.0 Overcoming gravity for sitting	2.2 Using righting reactions for standing	2.4 Walking	2.6 Walking to a location	2.8 Grasping for stabilizing
Level 3: Manual Actions	3.0 Grasping objects	3.2 Distinguishing objects	3.4 Sustaining actions on objects	3.6 Noting effects of actions on objects	3.8 Using all objects
Level 4 Goal-directed Actions	4.0 Sequencing familiar actions	4.2 Differentiating features of objects	4.4 Completing a goal	4.6 Personalizing features of objects	4.8 Learning by rote memorization
Level 5: Exploratory Actions	5.0 Comparing and varying actions and objects	5.2 Discriminating sets of actions and objects	5.4 Self-directing learning	5.6 Considering social standards	5.8 Consulting with others
Level 6: Planned Actions	6.0 Planning actions				

Adapted from a supplemental educational handout by D. B. McCraith and C. A. Earhart, "Cognitive Disabilities Model: Theory, Assessment, and Intervention" for a workshop conducted by C. A. Earhart, D. B. McCraith, and L. Riska-Williams (May 2016), University Health Network, Toronto, Canada. Copyright © 2016, 2017 by Allen Cognitive Group/ACLS and LACLS Committee, Camarillo, CA. Permission required to duplicate, copy, or modify this table. Contact www.allencognitive.org.

Allen's levels and modes represent a truly occupational therapy contribution to other coma or cognitive scales such as the Glasgow Coma Scale and the Rancho Los Amigos Scale. The occupational therapy elements of function and doing can provide the occupational therapist with valuable information that can be used to plan treatment and appropriate treatment goals and to prepare for discharge.

(Note that client-centered theory and the Canadian Model of Occupational Performance [CMOP] are listed in the following section because client-centered intervention forms the basis for the CMOP).

The Person-Environment-Occupation Theory

Commonly referred to as P-E-O, this theory originated in Canada (Law, Cooper, Strong, Rigby, & Letts, 1996) (Box 5-4). Person-Enviornment-Occupation grew from the professional need to describe the theory and clinical application of the dynamic interactions among the person, the environment, and the occupation. The P-E-O is seen as a transaction between the interdependent person and the environment, which, in turn, affects the occupation (Law et al., 1996).

In this transactional model, no evaluation or screen is specifically aligned or suggested, as the evaluative or screening tool should be directly in line with the client in regard to age, stage, diagnosis, and setting (or environment).

BOX 5-3

SUMMARY OF FUNCTIONAL COGNITIVE ABILITIES AND INTERVENTION GUIDELINES FOR THE COGNITIVE LEVELS IN THE ALLEN COGNITIVE SCALE[a,b,c]

Cognitive Level	1 Automatic Actions	2 Postural Actions	3 Manual Actions	4 Goal-Directed Actions	5 Explortory Actions	6 Planned Actions
FUNCTIONAL COGNITIVE ABILITIES						
Sensory Cues Attended To	Subliminal cues	Proprioceptive cues	Tactile cues	Visible cues	Related cues	Symbolic cues
Motor Actions: Spontaneous Imitated	Automatic None	Postural Approximate	Manual Manipulations	Goal-directed Replications	Exploratory Novelty	Planned Unnecessary
Purpose/Intent	Arousal	Comfort	Interest	Compliance	Self-control	Reflection
Learning	Habituates to repeated sensory cue	Approximates demonstrated postural action	Imitates demonstrated manual action	Imitates demonstrated short sequence	Discovers novel solutions via trial and error	Infers, imagines potential novel solutions
Attention Span	Seconds	Minutes	Half Hours	Hours	Weeks	Past/Future

(continued)

Box 5-3 (CONTINUED)

SUMMARY OF FUNCTIONAL COGNITIVE ABILITIES AND INTERVENTION GUIDELINES FOR THE COGNITIVE LEVELS IN THE ALLEN COGNITIVE SCALE[a,b,c]

INTERVENTION GUIDELINES

OT Activities	Sensory stimulation	Gross motor exercise	Activities with repeated actions	Activities with several steps	Concrete activities	Conceptual activities
Teaching Methods	Introduce striking sensory cues on or in close proximity to body	Prompt or demonstrate postural actions in front of person	Prompt or demonstrate familiar repeated actions with safe objects	Provide exact samples; demonstrate situation-specific problem solving	Demonstrate new series of steps; provide short written directions; encourage exploratory problem solving	Consult, collaborate
ADL: Requires Assistance to	Initiate, complete tasks	Initiate, complete tasks	Initiate, set up, prompt familiar actions	Provide materials in familiar locations	Identify hazards	Provide resources
Safety: Requires Assistance to	Ensure intake, skin integrity	Prevent wandering, falls	Remove hazardous objects	Solve new problems	Issue warnings	Identify resources
Supervision Required	24 hour	24 hour	Frequent checks	Live alone with daily checks	Live alone with weekly checks	None

[a]Allen, C. (1985). Occupational Therapy for Psychiatric Diseases: Measurement and Management of Cognitive Disabilities. Boston, MA: Little, Brown, and Company, pp. 31-62; 82.

[b]Allen, C. K., Blue, T., & Earhart, C. A. (1995). Understanding cognitive performance modes. Ormond Beach, FLA: Allen Conferences.

[c]Earhart, C. A. (1992). Analysis of activities. In C. Allen, C. Earhart, & T. Blue. Occupational therapy treatment goals for the physically and cognitive disabled. Rockville, MD: AOTA, pp. 125-239.

Note: Adapted from a supplemental educational handout by C. A. Earhart for "Cognitive Disabilities Model: Theory, Assessment, and Intervention" by C. A. Earhart, D. McCraith, and L. Riska-Williams presented at a workshop on May 7-8, 2016 at the University Health Network, Toronto, Canada. Copyright © 2016, 2017, 2018 by Allen Cognitive Group/ACLS and LACLS Committee, Camarillo, CA. Permission required to duplicate, copy, or modify this table. Contact www.allencognitive.org.

The *person* is defined as "the unique being who assumes multiple roles and cannot be separated from context or situation." The person brings attributes, skills, knowledge, and experience to any situation (Law et al., 1996). In this case, the person is considered to be unique and different from any other person. Occupational roles assumed by the person differ and vary based on the degree of importance and the client's stage and chronological age (see developmental theory in this chapter for further information). Clients as individuals are continually changing and developing, so the therapist must take into account their level of motivation for this process. It

---

Box 5-4

Person-Environment-Occupation Concepts

The P-E-O represents three major components of occupational therapy's concepts of occupation. P represents the individual person, E represents the person's environment, and O represents the person's occupation. The greater the disparity among the person, the environment, and his or her occupation, the greater will be the challenge. However, if the person, environment, and occupation are closely aligned and overlap somewhat, this is considered to be a good fit for the client. If these three areas slightly overlap, the person, environment, and occupation facilitate progress and motivational confidence.

---

is important to consider culture, social and political etiquette and mores, and client responses. Frequently, client motivation and responses are guided by past successes and failures, the emotional situation (stability vs instability) of the client, client stress or anxiety, and the client's ability to focus on and attend to tasks. All of these considerations must be acknowledged because they affect occupational engagement and performance. (Law et al., 1996)

The *environment* is defined as "the context or situation where occupational performance takes place." The environment is further divided into the following subsets: culture, socioeconomics, the institution or facility, the physical situation, and the social situation. These subsets are considered to be horizontalized (i.e., they are all equally important). All aspects of the environment are constantly providing demands of and cues to the individual. (Law et al., 1996)

Occupation is defined as "self-directed and meaningful tasks and activities the person engages in throughout the life span." Occupations, including self-care, leisure, and productivity, are engaged in to satisfy an intrinsic need for self-maintenance, expression, and life satisfaction. Occupations are carried out through the various roles we assume during our day and throughout our life. When considering and looking at occupations, the focus should be on the characteristics of occupations or tasks, the degree of structure, the overall length of time of the occupation or activity, the level of complexity, and the task demands placed on the participant (Strong et al., 1999).

P-E-O theory takes into account occupations that are common to occupational therapy, as well as applications used by other disciplines, such as physical therapy or speech therapy. Because it is so variable, this theory can be used with a wide variety of clients with a variety of illnesses, injuries, or disabilities across the life span (Law et al., 1996).

The Kawa Model and Theory

Kawa is the Japanese word for "river." Consider the sides and bed of a river (the environment), rocks (life circumstances), and logs and driftwood (assets and liabilities), as well as everything else that might be in or part of a river. This model seeks to identify impediments and the fluidity of an individual's life progression through the metaphor of a river. The Kawa model considers all elements of a client's life—the social and cultural contexts, the conditions, elements, and components that may impede or facilitate one's life flow, both positive and negative. Occupational therapy intervenes to facilitate flow when the impediments of life (illness, injury, disability) obstruct flow patterns. The spaces through which the river water flows, or can flow, are representational of occupation or the "doing" process that is facilitated through occupational therapy.

The Kawa model represents the inclusion of an Eastern way of thinking about a theory, in contrast to the Western theories most occupational therapists are familiar with. Life in this model is described as a "complex, profound journey that flows through time and space like a river" (Iwama, 2002).

The Kawa model may seem to be a very different way of providing services from what is typical in a Western clinic setting. However, the overall concepts included in this approach serve as a metaphor for holistic, client-centered intervention. Its use of symbolism can be helpful when introducing clients to holism in evaluation and treatment, although I would suggest perhaps using at least one other Western-based theory to fortify services. This provides both a solid base for therapy as well as a means to visualize the flow of life for clients.

This approach also provides some food for thought and inspires creativity for treatment interventions, such as painting or drawing one's "personal river of life" and marking problem issues, the impediments that prevent the river flow, the culture and context of one's life, and so on. The Kawa model can be useful for reflecting and identifying issues and problems that impede and facilitate clients' progress in life; it also offers the opportunity for clients to identify what needs to happen to facilitate the flow of their life journey.

THEORIES FROM OUTSIDE OCCUPATIONAL THERAPY

The following theoretical bases were developed and researched by professionals outside of occupational therapy. These theories are, however, frequently used by occupational therapists in the clinical setting.

Developmental Theory

The developmental theory can be traced back to the "personal context" from the *Occupational Therapy Practice Framework* (OTPF; American Occupational Therapy Association [AOTA], 2012). How we function and move through our life more or less follows a sequence of events or developmental milestones (major events). The effect of illness, injury, or disability can be viewed through this developmental progression. It is no surprise that any illness, injury, or disability is reflected in the presence of development problems or issues. The overall effect of such concerns can help the therapist identify the effect of the illness, injury, or disability on the clients' abilities to function in their life occupations. It is therefore the role of the occupational therapist and other health care providers to view and address this discrepancy between clients' actual or chronological ages and their developmental ages. Additionally, the greater the discrepancy between chronological age and developmental age, the more serious the developmental lag is determined to be, and the more severe the problem. (Refer to Chapter 3 on pediatric occupational therapy for information on how to calculate chronological age.) Developmental age is usually calculated according to evaluation protocol. This developmental age is based on the clients' performance of evaluation items. The calculation for developmental age is specific to the evaluation performed by the therapist, although given client performance levels, the developmental age number should be relatively stable among any variety of evaluations the therapist selects for evaluation purposes. Once developmental age is calculated, one must determine what would be appropriate development for an individual of this age.

To do this, you must understand what is considered to be typical development versus abnormal development. In the case of a 5-year-old child, you would expect the child to be walking, talking, drawing or coloring, attending a preschool or educational program of some type, and playing both with other children and alone. Additionally, one would expect a 5-year-old to be self-feeding, doing most or all of the dressing, and independently toileting. Now, consider the problems that would be present if the person was chronologically 12 years old, but functioning at a 5-year-old developmental level; now consider what problems would be identified if the client were 25 years old with the same developmental skill set.

Many developmental theorists have described the developmental progression through life. Some notable theorists are Carl Jung (1914), Eric Erikson (1978), and, more recently, Laslett (1989) (Box 5-5).

Client-Centered Approach/The Canadian Model of Occupational Performance

The client-centered approach has evolved from the existentialism philosophies attributed to Rollo May, Irvin Yalom, and Eric Fromm and historically from Gabriel Marceau and Martin Buber. The existential philosophers were major contributors to the humanistic approach. Dr. Carl Rodgers and Abraham Maslow are considered to be major and more current contributors to the humanistic approach. Rodgers developed his client-centered approach based on the humanistic focus (and humanism is grounded and based in existentialism). Rogers felt that the client is the only real expert on his or her situation and formulated therapy based on salient information provided by the client. Maslow is noted for his Hierarchy of Needs; Maslow's pyramid indicates that basic needs must be met in the pyramid's escalating order for a person to be a functional and satisfied human being. One cannot move up the pyramid until basic needs, or foundational areas, are met (Box 5-6).

The AOTA has adopted client-centered practice as both a core value and as a component of the OTPF (AOTA, 2012). This was preceded by the Canadian Occupational Therapy Association's development and execution of client-centered practice (cited in Cole, 2012, p. 82) in the late 1980s and 1990s. This is best exemplified by the Canadian Occupational Performance Measure (Canadian Occupational Therapy Association, 1992), an interactional and client-centered evaluation in which the therapist asks or

Box 5-5

COMPARISON OF JUNG, ERIKSON, AND LASLETT

JUNG: SPIRITUAL DEVELOPMENT

- Birth to puberty: Blissful ignorance, inherited predispositions
- Puberty to 35 years: Conscious and doubting, taking on responsibility
- 35 years to old age: Change in direction to express latent part of self-individuation
- Infirmity and death: Infirmity, acceptance of death, afterlife, and collective unconscious

ERIKSON: PSYCHOSOCIAL DEVELOPMENT

- Birth to infancy: Trust vs mistrust
- 2 to 4 years: Autonomy vs shame and doubt
- 5 to 7 years: Initiative vs guilt
- 8 to 12 years: Industry vs inferiority
- 13 to 22 years: Identity vs role confusion
- 23 to 35 years: Intimacy vs isolation
- 35 to 50 years: Generativity vs stagnation
- 50 years to death: Integrity vs despair

LASLETT: FOUR AGES

- First: Childhood, dependency, socialization, education, little responsibility
- Second: Maturity, independence, family and social responsibility, earning a living
- Third: Retirement, crown of life, self-fulfillment, enjoying life for its own sake
- Fourth: Dependency, disengagement, frailty, preparing for death

Reprinted with permission from Cole, M. (2012). *Group dynamics in occupational therapy: The theoretical basis and practice application for group intervention* (4th ed.). Thorofare, NJ: SLACK Incorporated.

Box 5-6

HIERARCHY OF NEEDS

5. Self-actualization: The pinnacle of all human needs being met

4. Self-esteem: Feeling confident about one's self

3. Belonging and loving: Feeling a close and intimate connection with others

2. Safety needs: The sense of security and safety in one's life

1. Physiological needs: Health and wellness, adequate nutrition, housing

Cole, 2012

interviews the client concerning importance, satisfaction, and performance of functional areas of occupational therapy practice: self-care, work, and leisure. The client's responses form the basis for client-centered practice in occupational therapy. This represents a distinct departure from more traditional medical models of care and places the focus on what the client feels is important to his or her particular situation. When the client's information is interlaced with occupational therapy goals and interventions, a truly holistic, client-centered approach to therapy can be attained.

Psychodynamic Theory

This theory, formerly know as the *psychoanalytic approach,* can be attributed to Sigmund Freud and other psychiatrists and psychologists who practiced during late 19th and first half of the 20th century. Psychoanalysis was a widely accepted and highly regarded form of therapy, although few people understood the mechanics of this process. It has fallen out of favor in recent history for three reasons (Cole, 2012):

1. The process was lengthy.
2. Psychoanalysis was not researched-based.
3. The psychoanalysis process was expensive.

As the world has evolved, more realistic and outcome-oriented approaches have taken the forefront in the mental health domain. Psychoanalysis, although it continues to be practiced, has been replaced in most situations by active, talk, or action-oriented therapies. Additionally, the use of psychotropic medication (medications used to relieve or decrease the presence and persistence of psychiatric symptoms) are commonly prescribed by psychiatrists in lieu of psychoanalysis.

Historically, the psychodynamic approach can be traced back to Sigmund Freud, famously recognized as the "father of psychoanalysis," who conceived the concept of the psyche comprising three components: the id, ego, and superego. The id is viewed as the unconscious, biological, and primitive component that operates on the pleasure principle. Consider that the id is present in infants and that infants seek pleasure or gratification and will perform infantile actions to get what they want or need—cry, oppose, fuss, yell, or be inconsolable. The ego, the psychological component of the psyche, interacts with the external world and functions to maintain balance between the internal and external components. The ego bases actions on experience, seeking logical outcomes and compromising as necessary. The superego functions with the external world and is the social component of the psyche, representing the conscience and societal rules. It seeks idealism and perfection, and for this reason is frequently illogical and unrealistic.

Interventions using the psychodynamic approach work best with higher-functioning individuals. Cole (2012) indicated that group work using this approach deviates from more traditional methods of conducting groups because of the higher functioning cognitive status of the clients. Such work includes "brainstorming" and planning to make decisions about what needs to be done, how things will be accomplished, and who will be responsible for particular work assignments—the actual "doing" of the task and evaluation of how the task and group functioned. The types of activities that can be completed using this theory are varied and may include planning and

<table>
<tr><td>

BOX 5-7

BEHAVIORAL THERAPY GOALS

Behavioral goals follow a consistent structure that can be applied to any appropriate client task, from activities of daily living, cooking, and craft task involvement to driving, marital problems, or child care—and anything else a client may encounter. Behavioral goals are observable (you can see the goals being worked on or accomplished); behavioral goals are objective (whatever action is being performed either is or is not being performed); and behavioral goals are measurable (they are based on time duration, frequency, completion).

</td></tr>
</table>

cooking a meal; organizing a holiday event, party, or dance; or engaging in creative activities such as fine art, crafts, dance, drama, or music to accomplish group goals. Also, consider the complexity of activities such as these, and you will gain a greater understanding of the high-functioning level of clients involved with this type of theoretical approach.

Occupational therapy contributors to the use of the psychodynamic or psycho-analytic approach during the 1950s and 1960s include Gail Fidler and Ann Mosey.

Behavioral and Cognitive Theories

Behavioral Theories

Pure behaviorism considers modes of acting (or behaving) that are problematic for the client and others. Strict behaviorist methods, which are still applicable in practice today, include the use of behavioral goal writing, processes of chaining and shaping, conditioning and habits, reinforcement, rehearsal and practice, role-playing, and desensitization and biofeedback (Cole, 2012). The goals of behavioral therapy are described in Box 5-7.

The following paragraphs describe and define behavioral therapy concepts:

- Behavioral goals: Any good goal, and all behavioral goals, should meet the following criteria for evaluation: Is this observable? Is this measurable? Is this objective? For the purpose of good note-writing, it is also wise to include a time frame for the goal being met. These items make the behavioral goal objective, understandable, and easy to engage in therapy.

- Chaining: Consider the links in a chain or a necklace. Each link connects to the next link; once all the links are connected, a chain or necklace results. Therefore, chaining means that one action is intimately connected to the preceding and following action. Consider toothbrushing within this context. One must first select, then pick up the toothbrush, apply toothpaste, place the toothbrush with toothpaste on the teeth, move the toothbrush around inside the mouth making sure to brush each tooth, repeat this for any number of seconds, spit out the toothpaste, rinse the mouth, rinse the toothbrush, replace the toothbrush, and dry the outside of the mouth. If these steps are done out of sequence, the teeth will not get brushed or will be brushed incorrectly.

- Shaping: This term relates to approximating a desired behavior or action. Think of a blob you are trying to craft into a ball. Initially, the substance will have no form, but as you work on the material, you get closer and closer to the desired shape. Shaping is like this. In occupational therapy, you would work on task components by beginning more generally, then work more specifically until the action is accomplished. This is frequently confused with chaining. Remember that chaining represents distinct actions, whereas shaping involves working from more general to more specific tasks or behaviors.

- Conditioning and habits: Habits are actions we do so frequently that they become automatic. The action is generally taken to achieve a goal and runs the gamut of getting ready in the morning with activities of daily living to performing calculations in one's head. Conditioning can be defined and understood as the learning process each person experiences to attain something that is determined to be desirable or positive. Frequently, if one is conditioned, the action performed will become a habit.

- Reinforcement: Reinforcement of a desired behavior or action can be external (e.g., a stick of gum) or internal (e.g. the sense one gets from doing something nice for another person). Reinforcement is effective as a reward for clients, but the effect of the reinforcing mechanism weakens over time and must be changed. If an occupational therapist is working with a group of incarcerated youth, getting an additional 5 minutes of gym time may be effective for a while, but this will weaken over time. Perhaps the next reinforcing tool would be to increase both gym time and telephone or computer time. Overall, for any reinforcement to achieve the desired action, it must be meaningful to the individual, or it is not useful or beneficial.

- Rehearsal and practice: When dealing with behaviors and behavioral changes, rehearsing the desired behaviors, as occurs in assertiveness training, is necessary. This enables the client to rehearse how and what to do. By rehearsing and practicing new behaviors, the client can learn how to develop skills and actions that will be more positive and beneficial in life. One approach to working with clients is the biomechanical model. This model is frequently used in physical disability work in occupational therapy. The biomechanical model focuses on the increase of strength, range of motion, and endurance. For example, this model may be used with a client who has sustained a cerebrovascular accident. Practice of appropriate exercise, correct positioning of the affected limb or limbs, transferring from one surface to another surface, etc. require acquired skills. These tasks must be done correctly to maximize client progress. Therefore, practice of these actions is necessary.

Cognitive Theories

Cognition can be defined in many ways. According to Kielhofner (2010), cognition can be described as follows:

- The process of experiencing and engaging in the complexities of everyday life (Lazzarini, 2005 as cited in Kielhofner, 2010)

- The process by which sensory input is transformed, reduced, elaborated, reduced, stored, recorded, and used (Levy & Burns, 2005 as cited in Kielhofner, 2010)
- The capacity to take in, organize, assimilate, and integrate new information with previous experience and to adapt to environmental demands by using previously acquired information to plan and structure behavior for goal attainment (Toglia, 2005 as cited in Kielhofner, 2010)

Cole (2012) indicated that "most of the cognitive frames of reference in occupational therapy are derived from "learning theories that grew from the roots of behaviorism in the 1930s and 1940s." (p.155)

Because cognition figures constantly in our daily lives, imagine how a person who is experiencing cognitive problems deals with common, everyday tasks. For example, in the case of a client with Alzheimer's disease, as cognitive processes become impaired, the client's abilities to move through life consistently diminish. In someone who has experienced a traumatic brain injury, common, everyday tasks are no longer automatic or easily accessed. As one supervisor of mine said during my Fieldwork II experience (Amy Cowey, OTR/L, verbal communication, HealthSouth Harmarville, 1984), "the person may look the same, but the personality has changed, so they are a different person. This causes so many problems with loved ones." This statement is absolutely true.

For cognitive issues, one screen—the Mini-Mental State Exam—provides the therapist or health care provider with a quick and simple way to assess cognition. The screen includes questions related to client orientation (name, day, season), the ability to perform simple calculations, spelling, memory, and drawing simple and overlapping shapes, among other items. It takes only a few minutes to complete, is easily scored, and provides the therapist with a general sense of how the client is functioning in regard to cognitive processes (National Center for Biotechnology Information, 2005).

This screen might be followed by Joan Toglia's Contextual Memory assessment (Toglia, 1993), which includes immediate and recent memory recall of pictures (activities of daily living or restaurant pictures) using both a context ("think of your daily morning routine," i.e., developing a story as a means to remember) and non-context (not developing a story but being asked to look at 20 pictures). When dealing with cognitive problems, the therapist assesses immediate then recent (things that have occurred in the past 20 minutes) memory. This relates to clients looking at 20 pictures and to answering questions about how they think their memory is in regard to their past memory abilities; that is, they assess their memory skills in a client-centered manner.

For example, clients with Alzheimer's disease may remember their first date but cannot remember what they had for lunch today. Additionally, clients may experience inconsistent memory in which they remember, for example, what work they did and be able to execute some basic work tasks but may not remember the names of family members or loved ones. These types of memory problems provide challenging situations for clients, therapists, and significant others.

What do occupational therapy interventions look like using behavioral and cognitive theories? A wide variety of physical, creative, and social-recreational activities can be used when working with these theories. It is best to consider the client's age because the therapist would want to formulate interventions that have "just the right fit"—not too difficult and not too easy. It is also important to consider safety issues, the spatial environment, and lighting to promote optimal client performance. Clients' diagnosis are also crucial to consider when selecting intervention activities. If behavior or cognitive issues are of primary importance to clients, activities that promote engagement, repetition, and learning will increase the likelihood that the clients will participate in and enjoy the task.

SUMMARY

Theory provides the practitioner with a structure for practice, along with a way of thinking about evaluation and intervention. Theory substantiates the what, why, where, when, and how of the services we provide to a given client. A basic understanding of the various theories is important, as is gaining an understanding of the types, ages, and stages of clients we work with, to select or frame our evaluation and interventions based in the correct theory. Recognize that some theories are general in nature, and other theories are more specific and focused on particular issues.

QUESTIONS TO CONSIDER FOR STUDENT LEARNING AND REASONING

1. As a newly graduated occupational therapy student, you realize that your client has never participated in many daily activities that are considered age-appropriate or attained the skills to do so. Will you rehabilitate or habilitate this client, and why?

2. A divorced and depressed individual says, "I can't do things with my married friends, and I don't have any single friends. Because of this, I just stay home and feel bad about the direction my life has taken. I used to love to go to movies, go out to dinner, and go for long walks. Now, I just feel like everyone is looking at me because I'm alone." What theory might support the development and refinement of leisure skills, along with bolstering the ability to deal with the feedback or comments of others? What components of this theory would substantiate its use in this situation?

3. Most of the clients who comprise your caseload are at least 10 to 20 years older than you are. How can you establish a solid and professional relationship with these individuals, and what approach will help you in the development of this relationship? In what ways will this theoretical approach help you?

4. Consider two very different client groups: Group A includes individuals who have not attained developmental milestones and clients who are sensory defensive, especially with tactile or touch issues; group B includes adults who want to create items to sell for fundraising initiatives. The activity that is determined to be appropriate for both groups is baking cookies. First, what theories supplement working with each group (the theories will be quite different). Second, how could you adapt making cookies with these two very different client groups? Third, how do your identified theories support your group activity with these clients?

REFERENCES

Allen, C. (1997). Allen's cognitive levels. Allen Conference Materials.

American Occupational Therapy Association. (2012). Occupational Therapy Practice Framework: Domain & process. *American Journal of Occupational Therapy, 62*, 635–682.

Brown, C., & Dunn, W. (2002). *The Sensory Profile: Adolescent and adult*. New York, NY: Pearson.

Brainy Quotes (2018). Piaget Quotes on Childhood Play. Retrieved from: http://www.brainyquotes. Piaget./play.com

Canadian Association of Occupational Therapy. (1992). *The Canadian Occupational Performance Measure*. Toronto, Canada: Author.

Cole, M. (2012). *Group dynamics in occupational therapy: The theoretical basis and practice application for group intervention* (4th ed.). Thorofare, NJ: SLACK Incorporated.

Collins Dictionary. (2018). Definition of frame of reference. Available from: www.collinsdictionary.com/defintion/frameofreference

Dunbar, S. (2007). Theory, frame of reference, and model: A differentiation for practice consideration. In S. Dunbar (Ed.), *Occupational therapy models for intervention with children and families*. Thorofare, NJ: SLACK Incorporated.

Erikson, E. H. (1978). *Adulthood*. New York, NY: Norton.

Frank, J.D. (1958). The therapeutic use of self. *American Journal of Occupational Therapy*. July-August, 12, 4, 215-225.

Hoffart, N., & Woods, C. Q. (1996). Elements of the nursing professional practice model. *Journal of Professional Nursing, 12*, 354–364.

Iwana, M. (2002). *The Kawa model: Culturally relevant occupational therapy*. New York, NY: Elsevier/Churchill Livingstone.

Jung, C. G. (1914). *On Psychological Understanding. In Collected Works 3*. Princeton, NJ: Princeton University Press.

Kielhofner, G. (2009). *Conceptual foundation of occupational therapy practice* (4th ed.). Philadelphia, PA: F.A. Davis.

Kielhofner, G., & Burke, J. (1980). A model of human occupation, part 4. Assessment and intervention. *American Journal of Occupational Therapy, 34*, 777–788.

Laslett, P. (1989). *A Fresh Map of Life: The Emergence of the Third Age*. Cambridge, MA: Harvard University Press.

Law, M., Cooper, B., Strong, S., Rigby, P., & Letts, L. (1996). The person–environment–occupation model: A transactive approach to occupational performance. *Canadian Journal of Occupational Therapy, 63*, 9–23.

Lazzarini, I. (2005). A nonlinear approach to cognition: A web of ability and disability. In N. Katz (Ed.), *Cognition and occupation across the lifespan: Models for intervention in occupational therapy* (2nd ed.). Bethesda, MD: AOTA Press.

Levy, I., & Burns, T. (2005). Cognitive disabilities reconsidered: Implications for occupational therapy practitioners. In N. Katz (Ed.), *Cognition and occupation across the lifespan: Models for intervention in occupational therapy* (2nd ed.). Bethesda, MD: AOTA Press.

Merriam Webster Dictionary. (2018). Definition of approach. Retrieved from: https://www.merriam-webster.com/dictionary/approach

National Center for Biotechnology Information. (2005). Mini-Mental State Examination. Retrieved from https://www.ncbi.nlm.nih.gov/projects/gap/cgi-bin/GetPdf.cgi?id=phd001525.1

Oxford Dictionary, (2018). Definition of theory. Retrieved from: www.oxforddictionaries.com/definition/theory

Punwar, A. (1996). *Introduction to occupational therapy.* Philadelphia, PA: Lippincott, Williams, and Wilkins.

Reed, K., & Sanderson, S. (1999). *Concepts of occupational therapy* (4th ed.). Philadelphia, PA: Lippincott, Williams, & Wilkins.

Sensory Integration Global Network (SIGN). (2018.) Sensory integration theory (definition). Retrieved from: http://www.siglobalnetwork.org

Strong, S., Rigby, P., Stewart, D., Law, M., Letts, L., & Cooper, B. (1999). Application of the Person-Environment–Occupation Model: A practical tool. *Canadian Journal of Occupational Therapy, 66,* 122–133.

Taylor, R. (2008). *The intentional relationship: Occupational therapy and use of self.* Philadelphia, PA: F.A. Davis.

Toglia, J. (1993). Contextual Memory Test. https://trove.nla.gov.au/work/31633376?q&version Id=38350475+47569024

Toglia, J. (2005). A dynamic interactional approach to cognitive rehabilitation. In N. Katz (Ed.), *Cognition and occupation across the lifespan: Models for intervention in occupational therapy* (2nd ed.). Bethesda, MD: AOTA Press.

Legislation and Its Effect on Current Occupational Therapy Practice
The Past 60 Years

KEY WORDS

- Americans with Disabilities Act (ADA)
- Consolidated Omnibus Budget Reconciliation Act (COBRA)
- Diagnosis-Related Group (DRG)
- Health Information Portability and Accountability Act (HIPAA)
- Health maintenance organization (HMO)
- Medical model
- Sick role

Hattjar, B.
Fundamentals of Occupational Therapy:
An Introduction to the Profession (pp. 93-104).
© 2019 Taylor & Francis Group.

This chapter provides a general, although not exhaustive, review of legislation and legislative endeavors that have served to shape the face of the profession. The world of 1954 was radically different from that of today. Imagine living in a world where there was no Internet, no cell phones, no social media, and no diversity and inclusion components to health care. The traditional "medical model" was considered to be the gold standard. Health care in the United States was considered to be among the best in the world. It usually took place in a hospital or doctor's office. Health care, during that time, focused on the amelioration of illness, injury, or disease. The patient—not "client"—was considered to be "sick," and the health care provider made choices for the patient (see Chapter 2, Box 2-2 for information on the *sick role*).

In the 1950s, polio had just been eradicated with the Salk vaccine, and Thorazine (chlorpromazine) became readily accessible for the treatment of psychosis. Occupational therapy was not a clearly understood or known entity in health care. In fact, it was not until the mid- to late-1950s that the profession addressed the shortage of professional-level practitioners and transitioned into the developmental of the technical level, the certified occupational therapy assistant (COTA).

Through increasing the sheer number of occupational therapy practitioners, the division of the professional (registered occupational therapist, or OTR) and technical (COTA) levels of the profession, and attempting to define the profession and the scope of the profession, a clearer understanding of the breadth of occupational therapy was better able to be communicated and evidenced to members of other health care professionals and to the patients/clients served by occupational therapy.

The 1960s was a time of social and cultural unrest. The passage of the Civil Rights Amendment and of Medicare and Medicaid legislation addressed some cultural and social issues that pervaded this decade. The situations and needs of people outside of mainstream America were being acknowledged.

The 1970s continued to be a period of unrest. During this decade, the Equal Rights Amendment was passed, along with the beginning of health care disparity and the development and increased use of health maintenance organizations (HMOs) as opposed to more traditional health care options. Disparity in health care has been a societal and cultural issue since the United States began to offer, then deal with health care issues. However, disparity that became acknowledged in the 1970's was more obvious due to media coverage, public awareness of the have and have-not populations, and the fact that individuals were speaking up and questioning what was wrong with health care in the United States This was done to avert high costs and physician specializations and to promote better and certainly more affordable health care for U.S. citizens.

In 1972, President Richard Nixon increased payments for workers who had been injured in the work setting. Before this time, people who sustained a work-related injury received compensation benefits that placed them at the poverty line or below. President Nixon and Congress placed a "new minimum" compensation payment of approximately 60% of gross wages or 80% of net wages. Once this compensation hike became law, the number of workers compensation cases substantially increased. This, in turn, led to the conceptualization and subsequent development of "work-hardening" programs, which were designed to simulate work and minimize the number of lost-wage days (Matheson, 1990).

In 1973, the Rehabilitation Act provided for nondiscrimination of qualified individuals based on their disability. A disability no longer could disqualify someone from services or benefits. Equally qualified applicants were to be viewed as "equals" during the job application and hiring process. This legislation highlighted the need for worker accommodations, which, in turn, would later bring about the *Americans With Disabilities Act* (ADA). President Nixon supported this legislation, but because of the Watergate scandal, focus on the Rehabilitation Act was lost. President Jimmy Carter was a strong believer in the concepts included in the 1973 Rehabilitation Act during his term as president (1976-1980), but political unrest in the Middle East forced him to focus his attention on that situation.

The 1980s saw the creation of Diagnosis-Related Groups (DRGs), which limited the number of traditional in-hospital days and appropriate services for specific diagnostic groups. This created the upsurge of home care and lesser care facilities, both of which became large employers of occupational therapists and COTAs. DRGs decreased and then eliminated the "fee-for-service" system of health care payment. President Ronald Reagan was bombarded with skyrocketing health care costs, hence the enactment of DRGs and the increase in HMOs and incentives for medical students to generalize rather than specialize in practice focuses.

President George H. W. Bush enacted the ADA in 1990, placing the needs of the disabled population at the forefront of society. Cost containment became a major problem in the 1990s, and capitation of billable services for occupational therapy, physical therapy, and speech-language pathology occurred in 1998 (Box 6-1). This posed employment problems for occupational therapists, and many jobs were lost. However, with every cloud comes a silver lining: occupational therapists began to develop new or emerging areas of practice, including driving skills, vision, and some mental health initiatives. At the beginning of the 21st century, many of these emerging areas became standard practice or specialty practice areas. These areas served not only to expand the practice base, but also promoted a more holistic and less traditional view of the profession. This expansion continues today.

In 1996, the *Healthcare Information Portability and Accountability Act* (HIPAA) was passed. This ensured, among other things, the confidentiality of patient health information, both hard copy or electronic medical records. The privacy of patient/client records and the sharing of a person's medical information considered privacy, accessibility to information, and how information could safely be shared through levels of protection such as electronic encryption, codes, and passwords, along with employee education. This protective approach continues today. This represented a marked change in health care insurance and within the health care industry. These changes also promoted legislative bickering in the political arena where some legislators and members of our government supported the Affordable Care Act (ACA) concepts and other individuals did not support these changes.

The early decades of the 21st century saw the dawn of the ACA. The ACA seeks to provide health care coverage continuity for all Americans. It covers a variety of circumstances that affect Americans throughout the life span.

Box 6-1

MAKING LEMONADE OUT OF LEMONS

Capitation of charges to Medicare in 1998 forced many health care providers in occupational, physical, and speech therapies out of their jobs. This "cap" for billing charges included an annual billable aggregate (total) billing fee for occupational therapy of $1500 annually, whereas the annual aggregate billing fee for physical and speech therapy *combined* was $1500. If you consider that an evaluation charge and treatment session costs could mount up quickly, it is easier to understand how job losses could occur. Because services could not be billed through insurance once a client had "maxed out," any further treatment expenses had to be paid out of pocket. Medicare is usually the major source of health insurance for those over age 65 years—people who are retired and living on a fixed income—so assuming the burden of additional expenses for therapy services was difficult or impossible for many clients. Therefore, clients did without needed services. This situation was rectified in the first decade of the 21st century. However, during this time of flux, creative occupational therapists chose to "make lemonade out of lemons" and developed "service niches."

During the late 1990s and early into the 21st century, occupational therapists began to get involved in areas that are now considered to be specialty or best practice (widely accepted and understood practice) areas including low vision, driving, ergonomics and work, and private practice businesses, to name a few. Some of these areas are still developing, whereas other areas are well-established. This situation nevertheless represents the determination and creativity of occupational therapists. In these niches, therapists either performed services and billed services to clients (out-of-pocket expenses) or became aligned with business or industries that supported the services, such as driving schools, physicians specializing in low vision, or businesses or industries with high numbers of worker injuries.

Legislation for health care initiatives was enacted in the past but was not as all encompassing and consistent as it has become during the past few decades. During the mid- to late-20th century, the United States appeared to have one of the best health care systems in the world. This has declined over recent decades due to the escalating costs of health care, the increasing numbers of underinsured or unin-sured people, and the fact that we are living longer due to medical advancements. Superimpose the aging baby boomer generation on all of this, and this is where the United States is as this book goes to press: we are in a state of flux, and the future of our health care system is in question.

As a student new to the profession, it is important to understand the effects and influence of major legislation on health care and on the profession of occupational therapy. This chapter is not inclusive of all legislation enacted during the past 60 years, but rather is a general review of how more wide-scope legislation enacted and revised has affected our profession. This is crucially important for students to under-stand because the legislative initiatives included in this chapter have molded our profession, and all health care professions, into what they are today and will continue to do so in the early decades of the 21st century. The years provided in this section should help the student to draw a line between one generational point to the next.

1950 TO 1960

1954

Public Law (P.L.) 83-565: Vocational Rehabilitation Act Amendments (Hill-Burton Amendments) where medical and vocational services for individuals were highlighted, as these areas had not been explicitly addressed before. This represents an update to P.L. 78-133, the Vocational Rehabilitation Act Amendments (Barden-LaFollette Act of 1945). The 1945 act identifies the provision of medical services and vocational rehabilitation. Coverage was expanded to include services to visually impaired people and those with mental health problems or who were intellectually challenged. The 1954 act expanded service provision to include training of professional rehabilitation service providers (Reed, 1992).

1960 TO 1970

1963

President John F. Kennedy was instrumental in moving forward the Community Mental Health Act (also known as the *Mental Retardation and Community Mental Health Centers Construction Act of 1963*). This act altered the location of service delivery for individuals with mental health and intellectual development problems (then referred to as *mental retardation*) and diagnosis. Before this law was enacted, most services were delivered in hospital and/or residential settings. This law established comprehensive community mental health centers throughout the United States. This law served to close large inpatient or residential facilities and move the residents of these programs into the community. Along with this, the use of more and different psychotropic drugs and the institution of new, more current types of psychotherapy were also supported and suggested for community-based case. During the late 1950s and early 1960s, inclusion in the community was viewed as the most feasible solution for both mental health and intellectual disability problems (National Council for Behavioral Health, 2018).

1964

President Lyndon Johnson signed the Civil Rights Act of 1964. This act prohibits discrimination based on race, color, religion, or national origin. The spirit of this law is broad, but includes components like equal voting rights, prohibits segregation or discrimination based on race, color, religion, or national origin. It is broadly interpreted as "equal rights for all" although the concept of equal rights continues to be disputed to this day. Enactment of the Civil Rights Act is considered to be the most important piece of legislation in the past 100 years (Encyclopedia Britannica, 2018).

Title II of the Civil Rights Act prohibits discrimination in places of public accommodation because of race, color, religion, or national origin. Places of public accommodation are hotels, motels, restaurants, movie theaters, stadiums, and concert halls. Title III of the Civil Rights Act of 1964 prohibits discrimination in public facilities because of race, color, religion, or national origin. Public facilities are facilities owned, operated, or managed by state or local governments, such as court houses or jails (Findlaw, 2014).

1965

President Johnson signed the Medicare and Medicaid Ammendments to the Social Security Act. Medicare provides health care for people over age 65 years, or of retirement age. Medicaid provides health care for those living in poverty. Both older Americans and those living in poverty represented high-risk and noninsured components of the U.S. population. The intent of both of these acts was to end health care inequity and provide care for those who need it most.

Medicare is divided into Medicare Part A and Medicare Part B. Medicare Part A provides insurance for in-hospital, inpatient care including critical care units and hospitals and skilled nursing facilities (not custodial or long-term care facilities). It also covers hospice care and some home care. Medicare Part B covers doctors' services and outpatient facility care. Part B also covers some other medical services including that of occupational and physical therapists and home care. Part B helps to pay for these services and supplies when they are deemed to be medically necessary (Centers for Medicare & Medicaid Services, 2014). This usually requires that the treating therapies provide monthly updates to determine whether services are medically necessary. Although not a part of the original spirit of this act, prescription drug coverage for Medicare (Medicare Part D) recipients began on January 1, 2006. Medicare prescription drug coverage is likened to insurance that medications will be affordable, accessible, and may help to prevent escalating drug prices in the future. Most people will pay a fee for coverage because coverage is provided through private companies, not the government (Centers for Medicare & Medicaid Services, 2014). The fourth part of the Medicare quadrant, Medicare Part C, covers long-term care situations. For additional information, visit http://www.Medicare.gov.

1970 TO 1980

1973

Section 504 of the Rehabilitation Act of 1973 protects qualified individuals from discrimination based on their disabilities. In relation to work, qualified individuals with disabilities are defined as persons who, with reasonable accommodation, can perform the essential job functions for which they have applied or have been hired to perform. Reasonable accommodation means an employer is required to take reasonable steps to accommodate the disability unless it would cause the employer undue hardship (U.S. Department of Health & Human Services, 2006). In the case of this law, *disabilities* are defined as physical or mental impairments that substantially limit one or more life activities. People who have a history of or who are currently regarded as having a physical or mental impairment that substantially limits one or more life activities are also covered. Major life activities include caring for oneself, walking, seeing, hearing, speaking, breathing, working, performing manual tasks, and learning. Some examples of the impairments that may substantially limit major life activities, even with the help of medications or aids and devices, are AIDS, alcoholism, blindness or visual impairment, cancer, deafness or hearing impairments, diabetes, drug addiction, heart disease, and mental illness (U.S. Department of Health & Human Services, 2006).

1975

Public Law 94-142: The four purposes of PL 94-142 include (a) to ensure that all children with disabilities have available to them a free, appropriate public education that emphasizes special education and related services designed to meet their unique needs; (b) to ensure that the rights of children with disabilities and their parents (or caregivers) are protected; (c) to assist states and localities to provide for the education of all children with disabilities; and (d) to assess and ensure the effectiveness of efforts to educate all children with disabilities as a means to provide for educational equity (U.S. Department of Education, 2010).

1980 TO 1990

1986

Consolidated Omnibus Budget Reconciliation Act (COBRA) made moving from one job to another less difficult because health insurance and health care options could be retained by the individual. It gives workers who lose their benefits the right to continue group health benefits provided by their employer, which they pay for out of pocket. COBRA applies not only to job changes but also in any of the following cases: voluntary or involuntary termination of the covered employee's employment for reasons other than gross misconduct; reduced work hours of the employee; the covered employee becomes entitled to Medicare; divorce or legal separation of the covered employee; death of the covered employee; and loss of dependent child status as identified under plan rules of the employer (Healthcare.gov, 2018). COBRA occurs for a specified period of time depending on the reason for losing health coverage.

DRG's came onto the health care scene in 1986 as a means of decreasing health care costs for hospital length of stays. DRG's identified a schedule and structure for the patient length of stay for specific diagnosis groups. The introduction of DRG's was radically different from previous "fee for service" plans. Fee for service means that a health care provider could and would bill for a specific service, like an office visits, bloodwork tests, or a therapy evaluation and receive payment for that particular service. Retrospectively, in 1983 Medicare's Prospective Payment Service (PPS) became effective in 1500 hospitals. By 1984, the number of hospitals using the PPS system grew to more than 3500. PPS was deemed necessary to avert continued escalation of health care costs (Mistichelli, 1984). Medicare costs had risen 19% annually from 1979 through 1983. To prevent acceleration of Medicare costs, DRGs classified 467 illness categories, and PPS replaced the previously used "fee-for-service" plan. In 1986, DRGs set the acceptable length of stay for specific diagnosis groups. Extension of care for a client could be applied for, but usually clients were referred to lesser care units, facilities, or environments. Over time, this decreased the number of necessary in-hospital beds but increased the utilization of services in other areas such as nursing homes, assisted living facilities, skilled nursing units, home care, outpatient facilities, and hospice.

1990 TO 2000

1990

The ADA of 1990 prohibits discrimination and ensures that persons with disabilities have the same opportunities as everyone else to participate in daily life, including work, the purchase of goods and services, mobility in the home and community, and the ability to utilize and access state and local government and services (ADA. gov, n.d.). The profession of occupational therapy is a good fit with this law based on the breadth and scope of our profession. The ADA provides practical solutions to "accessibility" in the work arena, the outside world, and services and goods that nondisabled people can access. In essence, the ADA leveled the playing field for disabled populations and has promoted a better and more autonomous quality of day-to-day life for people with disabilities or who require accommodations.

1996

As noted earlier, the 1996 HIPAA provides for medical record and information confidentiality, including both hard copy and electronic transmission of patient information.

HIPAA originally only included the first two objectives, but has been expanded to include five total listed:

1. To ensure that people would be able to maintain their health insurance between jobs. This is the portability aspect of the act and has been successfully implemented.
2. The accountability section of the act is designed to ensure the security and confidentiality of patient information data. It also mandates uniform standards for electronic data transmission of administrative and financial data relating to patient health information.
3. Tax related health provisions dealing with certain deductions and other changes to health care laws as applicable.

4. Application and enforcement of group health plan requirements including changes for preexisting conditions and insurance coverage modifications or changes.

5. This title relates to company life insurance, the loss of insurance for people who lose U.S. citizenship for tax purposes, and financial rules and responsibilities for the company (CA.gov, 2018).

With the advance of technology and electronic information dissemination, HIPAA has modified and clarified how data can be transmitted, creating greater assurance of confidentiality and security.

2000 TO PRESENT

2014

The ACA is described as a vehicle to put consumers back in charge of their health care. The "Patient's Bill of Rights" under the ACA includes:

- Ending preexisting condition exclusions for children: Health plans can no longer limit or deny benefits to children under 19 years of age due to a preexisting condition.
- Maintaining coverage for young adults: Those under age 26 years may qualify for coverage under a parent's health care plan.
- Ending arbitrary withdrawals of insurance coverage: Coverage cannot be cancelled if an honest mistake was made.
- Guaranteeing the right to appeal: The patient has the right to request reconsideration of a claim if it was denied by the insurance company.

Because cost containment is important in the current health care arena, the ACA seeks to do the following:

- Lifetime limits on new health care plans are banned.
- Insurance companies must publicly justify any unreasonable rate increases.
- Insurance dollars must be spent on health care, not on administrative costs.

The ACA also promotes the following "care" items including:

- Preventative care will occur at no cost to the individual with no copayment.
- The individual can select a primary physician from a list of policy network physicians.
- In the case of an emergency, individuals can secure care both inside and outside of their network of providers (U.S. Department of Health & Human Services, 2017).

The future of health care in the United States is uncertain. The ACA continues to be legislatively disputed and other health care options are discussed but not mandated. The effect of the Baby Boomer generation reaching retirement age and the effect of this on Social Security, Medicare, and Medicaid is a legislative concern, although many boomers are working longer than the more typical "retirement at age

65" option that has been a part of our history in the United States. More individuals with diseases like cancer are experiencing a longer life due to developments in medicine and medications or treatments proving to be effective on extending life and the quality of life. More children are being diagnosed with mental health problems like autism spectrum disorder and genetic issues thus placing needs for treatment interventions and a lifelong strain on the health care system. Many or all of these issues will provide employment opportunities for occupational therapy services, the need for accredited education in the field, and the option for increasing employment needs within the profession. As occupational therapy students, you must keep abreast of these situations because not only will it affect your professional practice, but you may experience personal ramifications as they affect you and your loved ones.

LICENSURE AND REGISTRATION FOR OCCUPATIONAL THERAPY

Although licensure is not a federal edict, states regulate the provision of occupational therapy through licensure legislation. Licensure for occupational therapists began to gain momentum during the 1970s. State licensure ensures the public that people who refer to themselves as *occupational therapists* or *occupational therapy assistants* and who provide occupational therapy services are, in fact, entitled to use this title due to their education at an accredited occupational academic program (per the Accreditation Council for Occupational Therapy Education, or ACOTE) and completion of clinical fieldwork placements, the passing of a national certification test (the National Board of Certification for Occupational Therapists, or NBCOT), along with an extensive background checks for child abuse and criminal activity and finger printing.

The American Occupational Therapy Association (AOTA) (n.d.) states: Occupational Therapy is regulated in all 50 states, the District of Columbia, Puerto Rico, and Guam. Different states have different types of regulation that range from licensure, the strongest form of regulation, to title protection or trademark law, the weakest form of regulation. The major purpose of regulation is to protect consumers in a state or jurisdiction from unqualified or unscrupulous practitioners.

Licensure and supporting licensure requirements (e.g., continuing education requirements, cost, license renewal date) vary from state to state. To practice in your geographic location of choice, you must be licensed to practice in that state. In the case of being licensed in one state but moving to another, reciprocity exists. Reciprocity means that a license secured in one state is recognized by another. However, if you plan to practice in the state where you are moving, you must apply for application for licensure in that state, usually within a 30-day period from your date of residency. Many states also require a certain number of continuing education units (CEUs) in order to renew the license to practice occupational therapy.

OTR/L: These letters stand for "Occupational Therapist Registered" (registration with NBCOT). The "L" represents the letter used to identify licensure in a

---

Box 6-2

ACCREDITATION COUNCIL FOR OCCUPATIONAL THERAPY EDUCATION UPDATE

Per ACOTE, minimum educational preparedness will be changing by 2027. The entry level of practice for the OTR will be at the doctoral level. The entry level of practice for the COTA will be at the bachelor's degree level. Practitioners are expected to be "grandfathered in" at their current level of practice and education, so this does not represent job loss or replacement in the work situation.

---

particular state. Licensure requirements vary from state to state and include the 50 states plus the District of Columbia, Puerto Rico, and Guam (AOTA, 2018). Licensure insures the consumer that the consumer is protected from unscrupulous individuals Licensure must be renewed approximately every 2 years. The "R" means that the therapist is registered as an occupational therapist with the NBCOT. The "R" means that the therapist has passed the national certification examination that occurs after educational program graduation and satisfactory completion of clinical fieldwork placements. NBCOT requires ongoing CEUs for registration renewals every 5 years. This is important because of the ever-evolving health care arena. Participation in continuing education endeavors ensures that therapists are remaining current in their base of knowledge.

COTA/L: The COTA is subject to the same educational and certification/registration requirements as the occupational therapist. Additionally, the use of the "L" also represents licensure in the particular state or territory. NBCOT registration renewal is the same for the COTA, the technical level of occupational therapy practice.

SUMMARY

The extent and scope of legislation is broad and all-encompassing. The legislation identified reflects the composite of what makes up health care today. It is anticipated that health care, economic, and societal change and evolution will continue to influence legislation that reflects health care changes in the future. There currently is no certainty of where health care is going in the United States, but through our knowledge of past legislation, licensure laws in each state, and the securing of continuing education, occupational therapy practitioners can be assured of staying abreast and current in their knowledge and practice base (Box 6-2).

QUESTIONS TO CONSIDER
FOR STUDENT LEARNING AND REASONING

1. The legislation mentioned in this chapter has figured prominently in the clinical practice of occupational therapy. Select one piece of legislation and research it to determine how the law impacts an element of practice (like working in pediatrics, mental health, community practice, or physical disabilities).

2. How would one patient group be served by the legislation you have researched (from Question 1)? For example, if a piece of legislation mandates that community accessibility be addressed, like the addition of elevators in a building that had no elevators, what group of individuals would be best served by this addition?

3. Have any of the pieces of legislation identified in this chapter aided you or a loved one? Please identify the legislation and how it benefitted the person in question.

REFERENCES

ADA.gov. (n.d.). *Introduction to the ADA*. Retrieved from http://www.ada.gov/ada_intro.htm

American Occupational Therapy Association. (2018). Issues in licensure. Retrieved from https://www.aota.org/Advocacy-Policy/State-Policy/Licensure.aspx

California Department of Healthcare Services. (2018). *HIPAA Title Information*. Retrieved from: http://www.dhcs.ca.gov/formsandpubs/laws/hipaa/Pages/1.10HIPAATitleInformation.aspx

Centers for Medicare & Medicaid Services. (2014). *Medicare program: General information*. Retrieved from www.cms.gov/Medicare/Medicare-General-Information/MedicareGenInfo/Index.html

Encyclopedia Britannica. (2018). Civil Rights Act of 1964. Retrieved from: http://www.britannica.com

HealthCare.gov. (2018). *COBRA Definition*. Retrieved from: https://www.healthcare.gov/unemployed/cobra-coverage/

Hughes, J. (1994). *Approaches to the doctor–patient relationship*. Retrieved from http://www.changesurfer.com/Hth/DPReview.htm

Matheson, L. (1990). *The industrial rehabilitation certification workshop*. Keene, NH: Matheson Institute.

Mistichelli, J. (1984). *Diagnosis Related Groups*. Retrieved from https://repository.library.georgetown.edu/handle/10822/556896

National Council for Behavioral Health. (2018). *Community Mental Health Act*. Retrieved from https://www.thenationalcouncil.org/about/national-mental-health-association/overview/community-mental-health-act/

Reed, K. (1992). History of federal legislation for persons with disabilities. *American Journal of Occupational Therapy, 46*, 397–408.

Stiggelbout, A.M., Kiebart, G.M. (1997). A role for the sick role: Patient preferences regarding information and participation in clinical decision making. *Canadian Medical Association Journal (CMAJ), 157*(4),383-389.

U.S. Department of Education. (2010). Thirty-five years of progress in educating children with disabilities through IDEA. Retrieved from https://www2.ed.gov/about/offices/list/osers/idea35/history/idea-35-history.pdf

U.S. Department of Health and Human Services. (2006). *Fact sheet: Your rights under Section 504 of the Rehabilitation Act*. Retrieved from https://www.hhs.gov/sites/default/files/ocr/civilrights/resources/factsheets/504.pdf

U.S. Department of Health and Human Services. (2017). About the Affordable Care Act. Retrieved from http://www.hhs.gov/healthcare/rights

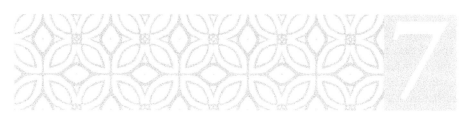

Trendsetters and Significant People in the Profession

KEY WORDS

- American Occupational Therapy Foundation (AOTF)
- *Centennial Vision*
- Eleanor Clarke Slagle Award
- Leaders and Legacies Society

Hattjar, B.
Fundamentals of Occupational Therapy:
An Introduction to the Profession (pp. 105-114).

Every profession has members who attain a degree of fame through their work. In occupational therapy, noted individuals such as Eleanor Clarke Slagle, Gail Fidler, Ann Mosey, Mary Reilly, Gary Kielhofner, Claudia Allen, and A. Jean Ayres, among others, are familiar to occupational therapy practitioners and educators for their professional contributions, theories, and evaluations. Their names have been referred to earlier in this textbook, and you will also see their names in many other textbooks.

Additionally, some occupational therapists have received the *Eleanor Clarke Slagle Award*, presented at the annual professional conference. This prestigious award is given to a professional member of the American Occupational Therapy Association (AOTA) who "has creatively contributed to the development of the body of knowledge of the profession through research, education, and/or clinical practice" (AOTA, 2018). Included in the receipt of this award at the AOTA annual national conference is the presentation of a motivating speech on a topic of interest to the recipient and to the professional body as a whole. Note that the presentation of the award occurs the year before the speech at the conference. The text of each speech is published in the *American Journal of Occupational Therapy* (AJOT). Later in the year, it is presented at the conference and usually in the last AJOT issue of the year (November/December) (Box 7-1).

What about some of the less recognizable names in occupational therapy who have contributed to and enhanced the profession? The intent of this chapter is to familiarize the student with people who have promoted and enhanced the profession with perhaps less fanfare or recognition than others have received. The contributions that therapists make to a profession are all important and significant, regardless of the level of professional or personal acknowledgment.

To equalize the selection of professionals for this chapter, I created a rubric for inclusion (Box 7-2). I also recognized the large number of people who might match rubric items and limited inclusion to only a few practitioners. It is up to the student to investigate and research other leaders who have made similar level contributions.

In alphabetical order, the following professionals were selected for inclusion:
- Charles H. Christiansen
- Winifred W. Dunn
- Karen Jacobs
- Fred Sammons
- Joan Toglia
- Renee Taylor

These leaders (cited with their professional and academic credentials) are recognized here for their professional contribution, and a brief history of their role as an occupational therapist is given. Also included is a structured text of their contributions within the context of the rubric. Note that some of the people have received the Eleanor Clarke Slagle Aware, and some have not.

BOX 7-1

ELEANOR CLARKE SLAGLE AWARD WINNERS (1955 TO 2019) AND PRESENTATION TOPICS

1955	Florence M. Stattell, "Equipment Designed for Occupational Therapy"
1956	June Sokolov, "Therapist Into Administrator: Ten Inspiring Years"
1957	Ruth W. Brunyate, "Powerful Levers in Little Common Things"
1958	Margaret S. Rood, "Every One Counts"
1959	Lillian S. Wegg, "The Essentials of Work Evaluation"
1960	Muriel Ellen Zimmerman, "Devices: Development and Direction"
1961	Mary Reilly, "Occupational Therapy Can Be One of the Great Ideas of 20th Century Medicine"
1962	Naida Ackley, "The Challenge of the Sixties"
1963	A. Jean Ayres, "The Development of Perceptual-Motor Activities: A Theoretical Basis for Treatment of Dysfunction"
1964	—
1965	Gail S. Fidler, "Learning as a Growth Process: A Conceptual Framework for Professional Education"
1966	Elizabeth June Yerxa, "Authentic Occupational Therapy"
1967	Wilma L. West, "Professional Responsibility in Times of Change"
1968	—
1969	Lela A. Llorens "Facilitating Growth and Development: The Promise of Occupational Therapy"
1970	—
1971	Geraldine Louise Finn, "The Occupational Therapist in Prevention Programs"
1972	Jerry A. Johnson, "Occupational Therapy: A Model for the Future"
1973	Alice Jantzen, "Academic Occupational Therapy: A Career Specialty"
1974	Mary Fiorentino, "Occupational Therapy: Realization to Activation"
1975	Josephine C. Moore, "Behavior, Bias, and the Limbic System"
1976	Joy A. Huss, "Touch With Care or a Caring Touch?"
1977	—
1978	Lorna Jean King, "Toward a Science of Adaptive Responses"
1979	Irene L. Hollis, "Remember?"
1980	Carolyn M. Baum, "Occupational Therapists Put Care in the Care System"
1981	—
1982	—
1983	Joan C. Rogers, "Clinical Reasoning: The Ethics, Science, and Art"

(continued)

	BOX 7-1 (CONTINUED)

ELEANOR CLARKE SLAGLE AWARD WINNERS (1955 TO 2019) AND PRESENTATION TOPICS

1984	Elnora M. Gilfoyle, "Transformation of a Profession"
1985	Anne Cronin Mosey, "A Monistic or a Pluralistic Approach to Professional Identity?"
1986	Kathlyn L. Reed, "Tools of Practice: Heritage or Baggage?"
1987	Claudia Kay Allen, "Activity: Occupational Therapy's Treatment Method"
1988	Anne Henderson, "Occupational Therapy Knowledge: From Practice to Theory"
1989	Shereen D. Farber, "Neuroscience and Occupational Therapy: Vital Connection"
1990	Susan B. Fine, "Resilience and Human Adaptability: Who Rises Above Adversity?"
1991	—
1992	—
1993	Florence A. Clark, "Occupation Embedded in a Real Life: Interweaving Occupational Science and Occupational Therapy"
1994	Ann P. Grady, "Building Inclusive Community: A Challenge for Occupational Therapy"
1995	Catherine Anne Trombly, "Occupation: Purposefulness and Meaningfulness as Therapeutic Mechanisms"
1996	David L. Nelson, "Why the Profession of Occupational Therapy Will Flourish in the 21st Century"
1997	—
1998	Anne G. Fisher, "Uniting Practice and Theory in an Occupational Therapy Framework"
1999	Charles H. Christensen, "Defining Lives: Occupation as Identity: An Essay on Competence, Coherence, and the Creation of Meaning"
2000	Margo B. Holmes, "Our Mandate for the New Millennium: Evidence-Based Practice"
2001	Winifred W. Dunn, "The Sensations of Everyday Life: Empirical, Theoretical, and Pragmatic Considerations"
2002	—
2003	Charlotte Brasic Royeen, "Chaotic Occupational Therapy: Collective Wisdom for a Complex Profession"
2004	Ruth Zemke, "Time, Space, and the Kaleidoscopes of Occupation"
2005	Suzanne M. Peloquin, "Embracing Our Ethos, Reclaiming Our Heart"
2006	Betty Risteen Hasselkaus, "The World of Everyday Occupation: Real People, Real Lives"
2007	Jim Hinojosa, "Becoming Innovators in an Era of Hyperchange"
2008	Wendy J. Coster, "Embracing Ambiguity: Facing the Challenges of Measurement"
2009	Kathleen Barker Schwartz, "Reclaiming Our Heritage: Connecting the Founding Vision With the Centennial Vision"
2010	Janice Burke, "What's Going on Here? Deconstructing Interactive Encounters"'

(continued)

	Box 7-1 (CONTINUED)

ELEANOR CLARKE SLAGLE AWARD WINNERS (1955 TO 2019) AND PRESENTATION TOPICS

2011	Beatriz C. Abreu, "Accentuate the Positive: Reflections on Empathetic Interpersonal Interaction"
2012	Karen Jacobs, "PromOTing Occupational Therapy: Words, Images, and Actions"
2013	Glen Gillen, "A Fork in the Road: An Occupational Hazard?"
2014	Maralynne D. Mitcham, "Education as Engine"
2015	Helen Cohen, "A Career in Inquiry"
2016	Susan L. Garber, "The Prepared Mind"
2017	Roger O. Smith, "Technology and Occupation: Past 100, Present and Next 100 Years"
2018	Gordan Muir Giles, not available at time of publication
2019	Ellen S. Cohn, not available at time of publication
AOTA, 2018	

Box 7-2

INCLUSION RUBRIC

1. The individual has made a noted contribution to the occupational therapy profession.
2. The individual exhibited or continues to exhibit ongoing motivation and productivity.
3. The contribution made by the individual have made a substantial difference within the profession and continue to do so through work and actions.
4. The contribution made by the individual represents a non–research-oriented contribution, although research may have become an element of his or her contribution.
5. The contribution made by the individual falls within the professional domain.
6. The contribution made by the individual may have originated within the realm of "emerging practice" but is, over time, considered to be a professional practice component or practice standard.
7. The contribution made by the individual supports AOTA's *Centennial Vision* for the profession of occupational therapy. The *Centennial Vision* for occupational therapy provided and continues to provide us with the overarching, nationwide, and global picture of where we are and where we need and want to move. It provides us with a structure and support for future professional—and personal—endeavors.

Box 7-3
THE AMERICAN OCCUPATIONAL THERAPY FOUNDATION: **VISION, MISSION, AND STRATEGIC GOALS**
THE VISION
"We envision a vibrant science that builds knowledge to support effective, evidence-based occupational therapy."
THE MISSION
"...to advance the science of occupational therapy to support people's full participation in meaningful life activities."
THE STRATEGIC GOALS
Research: To support initiatives that build research capacity and advance knowledge related to occupation, health, and well-being.
Sustainability: To develop the financial and human resources necessary to pursue the vision and mission of the Foundation.
Awareness: To increase public and professional recognition of AOTF and its purposes and activities.
AOTF, 2016b

Charles H. Christiansen, EdD, OTR/L, OT(C), FAOTA

After an extensive career of practice, research, administration, and professional promotion, Dr. Christensen retired in 2015. Throughout his career, he wrote extensively and was integral in the development and promotion of the occupational therapy *Centennial Vision* (AOTA, 2006) in the first decade of the millennium. One recent endeavor he embarked on was the promotion and development of the *American Occupational Therapy Foundation* (AOTF) *Leaders and Legacies Society* (Box 7-3). This society seeks to "identify, honor, and fully engage a cadre of occupational therapy professionals who have demonstrated their leadership abilities and skills through sustained service to the profession and wish to continue advancing the profession" (AOTF, 2015). As a leader in the profession, and a true and exemplary professional, Dr. Christiansen embodies the essence of the *Centennial Vision* of the profession.

Winifred W. Dunn, PhD, OTR/L, FAOTA

Dr. Dunn is a professor and chair of the Department of Occupational Therapy Education at the University of Kansas. She secured her master's degree in occupational therapy and special education from the University of Missouri. She attained her doctoral degree in applied neuroscience from the University of Kansas. Throughout her long career as an occupational therapist and occupational therapy educator, she has promoted the profession through numerous presentations nationally and internationally, and also through her writing and research. Her professional focus is on the effect of the senses in people's everyday lives, including infants, children, adolescents, and adults. She is the author/co author of the Sensory Profile and has updated and completed standardized research on the Sensory Profile 2. Her update ensures that practitioners will have the most current evidence to support their clinical decisions when using the Sensory Profile (Pearson Clinical, 2016).

In support of the *Centennial Vision*, Dr. Dunn has promoted the profession of occupational therapy and has furthered the use of assessment and screening tools (the Sensory Profile) to help practitioners tailor treatment interventions to an individual's sensory needs and issues. Her work has supported the use of and need for evidence on which to base practice.

Karen Jacobs, EdD, CPE, OTR/L, FAOTA

Dr. Jacobs's extensive body of work focuses on the "interface between the environment and human capabilities" (Boston University, 2016). This statement is significant because Dr. Jacobs has addressed the concept of work and task engagement from the perspectives of work, focus, cognition, and education. At the time of this writing, she is working on a 5-year research project, "Project Career: Development of an Interprofessional Demonstration to Support the Transition of Students With Traumatic Brain Injuries From Post-Secondary Education to Employment." She has, throughout her career, received numerous grants to support her research. She is also the founder of *WORK* journal, a publication that focuses solely on the publication of researched topics related to work issues. She has made numerous presentations on work-related topics throughout the United States, as well as internationally. She is a past president of the AOTA and has also received numerous professional awards based on her extensive body of work. She promotes the AOTA *Centennial Vision* through her combined work and promotion of occupational therapists creativity and professional spirit. Dr. Jacobs is currently is a clinical professor and director of Boston University's Online Post-professional Doctorate in Occupational Therapy (OTD) program.

Fred Sammons, PhD (Hon), OT, FAOTA

Although he began his career in teaching (mechanical drawing at the high school level), after serving in the Korean War, Dr. Sammons received his occupational therapy education at Virginia Commonwealth University. He began his clinical career as an occupational therapist at the Rehabilitation Institute of Chicago and assumed the department director position there from 1957 to 1960. At that time, he moved to the amputee clinic at Northwestern University. It was there that he began to design adaptive equipment and various items for amputees to enhance their daily lives. His creations met with an extremely positive response, so he began to design, manufacture, and distribute his devices full time in 1965. His company, Sammons, Inc., grew into a multimillion dollar company. It is now called Sammons-Preston, an AbilityOne Company. He has supported occupational therapy through grants, scholarships, and donations that support research. He is retired but continues to design adapted tricycles and bicycles for the American Business Clubs. The adapted tricycles and bicycles are given to people who have particular seating challenges (AOTF, 2016a). His love for design and product development has highlighted innovation and product use throughout the profession through the use of "adaptive equipment" items. His ability to develop a new business model for the profession serves to provide substantiation for other practitioners. His work supports the *Centennial Vision* and the concept of emerging practice through intent, focus, and the fruition of concepts and ideas—remember that occupational therapists are very creative and innovative! Dr. Sammons provides us with an exceptional role model for future endeavors.

Joan Toglia, PhD, OTR

With more than 30 years of experience in occupational therapy, Dr. Toglia is best known for her extensive work in cognitive rehabilitation theory and practice. In line with the *Centennial Vision*, her work has taken theoretical concepts and provided practitioners with practical and helpful applications. One of these is her Test of Contextual Memory. This test is aligned with her dynamic assessment and multicontextual approach (how an individual thinks about his or her thinking). Her work also encompasses evaluation and treatment for clients experiencing the effects of cognitive deficits, mild traumatic brain injury, self-awareness, right brain hemisphere dysfunction, nonverbal learning disability, spatial neglect, visuospatial deficits, and the rehabilitation of executive functioning (higher task abilities), and memory across the lifespan (Mercy College, 2016). Dr. Toglia has written and presented on numerous topics related to cognition. She is currently dean of the School of Natural Sciences at Mercy College, Dobbs Ferry, New York, where she was previously the program director of the Graduate Program in Occupational Therapy. Her skill in making cognitive concepts and cognitive rehabilitation a reality for many practitioners aligns with the *Centennial Vision* by promoting the occupational therapy profession and using innovative, practical means to provide purposeful and meaningful evaluations and interventions. Her body of work provides the health care professions with evidence of the effectiveness of occupational therapy.

Renee Taylor, PhD

Dr. Taylor, a professor of occupational therapy at the University of Illinois in Chicago, has also been affiliated with the Model of Human Occupation Clearinghouse since 2010 as the director. She is co-director of graduate studies with the PhD program in Kinesiology, Human Nutrition, and Rehabilitation Science and began her tenure in this position in 2008. She has been the principal investigator for federal research projects on chronic fatigue syndrome and served as a co-investigator on three other grants. Additionally, she has published more than 90 peer-reviewed articles on chronic fatigue and fibromyalgia (University of Illinois–Chicago, 2016).

In the occupational therapy realm, she has published books on the impact and power of the patient–therapist relationship, most notably *The Intentional Relationship: Occupational Therapy and the Use of Self* (Taylor, 2008). By writing about the impact of the patient–therapist relationship, this book, and the approach it describes, highlights the importance of the concept of "knowing" the self and the patient, understanding the therapeutic relationship on which we embark when we work with any client, and the occupational therapy precept of the power of both the task and the relationship formed with a client. Her current line of research focuses on supporting rehabilitation practice through the development and application of two conceptual practice models: Taylor's intentional relationship model and Dr. Gary Kielhofner's Model of Human Occupation (University of Illinois-Chicago, 2016). Through her ongoing research projects, the formulation of the intentional relationship model, and her ongoing work to promote a greater understanding of the psychological impact of health care, specifically occupational therapy, the profession gains substantiation for its presence and purpose in the current health care arena.

LEADERS AND LEGACIES SOCIETY

In 2014, the Leaders and Legacies Society initiated a founding membership cohort at the annual national AOTA conference. This honor was extended to members of the profession "whose work has made a difference in Occupational Therapy" (World Federation of Occupational Therapy, 2015). Membership is conferred in recognition of the significant service of these professionals and in acknowledgement of their ongoing desire to continue fostering the advancement of the occupational therapy profession (AOTA, 2014). Members inducted into this society represent individuals who, through leadership and professional work and passion, have contributed to the profession. The current president at the time of this writing, Ellen Kolodner (2017), stated in her portion of the keynote presentation at the 2017 Pennsylvania Occupational Therapy Conference that "our vision" for the profession is to promote "the telling of our own journey" in both personal and professional terms. In other words, occupational therapy provides each of us with professional and personal opportunities to lead and develop our own legacy. This leadership and legacy will influence the profession, our students, our clients, and the world of health care.

SUMMARY

As a student of occupational therapy, it is important to understand the network of individuals who have and continue to contribute to the profession. A professional contribution can come from local, state, or national involvement; research; quality clinical work; program or product development; writing; marketing; or mentoring. In other words, a professional contribution is really only limited by the type of work an individual therapist engages in on a professional level. The occupational therapy professionals identified in this textbook overall, and in this chapter specifically, provide examples of this very thing. As students in this profession, there is no one way to achieve your contribution to occupational therapy. Investigate, research, observe, listen, and engage in professional endeavors to discover how you can make your own mark on this remarkable profession. Always take the time to meet other practitioners, get to know and understand your professors, and learn from your clinical instructors to gain and acknowledge the contributions of occupational therapists. You will be amazed at what you learn.

QUESTIONS TO CONSIDER FOR STUDENT LEARNING AND REASONING

1. In your own words, identify why certain people were included in this chapter who might not normally be identified as "trendsetters" with the occupational therapy profession.
2. For each trendsetter mentioned in this chapter, name at least one contribution he or she has made to the body of knowledge for the occupational therapy profession.
3. This chapter begins by identifying individuals such as Eleanor Clark Slagle, Gail Fidler, Ann Mosey, Gary Kielhofner, Claudia Allen, and A. Jean Ayres. Research the names of these practitioners, and identify at least one contribution they made to the body of knowledge of the occupational therapy profession.

REFERENCES

American Occupational Therapy Foundation. (2018). *Honorary life member: Fred Sammons, PhD.* Retrieved from: www.aotf.org/Aboutaotf/Boardof Trustees/FredSammons
American Occupational Therapy Association. (2018). *The Eleanor Clark Slagle Lectureship award winners.* Retrieved from http://www.aota.org/education-careers/awards/recipients/eleanor-clarke-slagle-lectureship.aspx
American Occupational Therapy Foundation. (2016b). *Vision, mission and strategic goals.* Retrieved from http://www.aotf.org/aboutaotf/visionmissionstrategicplan
American Occupation Therapy Foundation. (2015). Leaders and Legacies Society: Making a Difference (brochure). Bethesda, MD: AOTA Press.
American Occupational Therapy Foundation. (2006). *AOTA's Centennial Vision.* Retrieved from https://www.aota.org/-/media/corporate/files/aboutaota/centennial/background/vision1.pdf
Boston University. (2016). *Karen Jacobs, EdD, CPE, OTR/L, FAOTA.* Retrieved from http://www.bu.edu/sargent/profile/karen-jacobs
Kolodner, E. (2017, October). Keynote presentation. Pennsylvania Occupational Therapy Association Annual Conference, State College, PA.
Leaders and Legacies Society. (2014). *Leaders and legacies society: Making a difference.* Bethesda, MD: AOTA Press.
Mercy College. (2016). *Joan Toglia PhD OTR.* Retrieved from http://www.taskstream.com/ts/toglia/Joan_Toglia
Pearson Clinical. (2018). Sensory Profile. Retrieved from http://www.pearsonclinical.com/therapy/products/100000822/sensory-profile-2.html
Taylor, R. (2008). *The intentional relationship: Occupational therapy and use of self.* Philadelphia, PA: F.A. Davis.
University of Illinois Chicago. (2018). College of Applied Health Sciences: Dr. Renee Taylor biography. Available from: http://www.ahs.uic.edu
World Federation of Occupational Therapy. (2015). *Leaders and legacies society brochure.* Bethesda, MD: AOTA Press.

Technology and Occupational Therapy

KEY WORDS

- Assistive technology
- High technology
- Home safety assessment (HSA)
- Low technology

Hattjar, B.
Fundamentals of Occupational Therapy:
An Introduction to the Profession (pp. 115-126).
© 2019 Taylor & Francis Group.

Technology, in general terms, is defined as "the application of scientific knowledge for practical purposes, especially in industry, machinery, and equipment." (Oxford Dictionaries, 2018). The term technology can mean different things to different people, although there is usually some reason or purpose for the use of technology.

In the case of, for example, technology in the work setting, training and analysis of the use of the technology can be a strong predictor of the actual usefulness of the item or process. For example, an office desk chair with cervical and lumbar support may be helpful in decreasing low back and neck strain, increasing worker comfort, and thereby increasing potential worker productivity. In the case of the individual, or for personal use (e.g., smart devices), education, training, practice, and repetition can ensure that the specific technology is used correctly and habitually. In this situation, the education and training of the potential user can make the difference between the device ending up unused or used frequently.

Humans have used technology throughout time. Prehistoric people learned how to create and control fire, and Neolithic people developed work and tools, thereby increasing their sources of food and protection through the use of available technology tools. Consider the building of the pyramids—an astounding, and perhaps confounding, achievement to this day—and temples. This displays the use of ancient technologies to support life and honor dignitaries, pharaohs, or the gods. The Romans built roads for travel and warfare, along with constructing an advanced system of aqueducts to support their supply of water. Boats and ships were built to aid in warfare and support the discovery of new lands. More recently, in the 1700s and 1800s, tool modification, food preservation techniques, and the development of items for warfare were considered technologically advanced. The discovery of electricity and the concepts of alternating and direct electrical currents lit up a world that was previously illuminated by gaslights, oil lamps, and candles. In the 20th century, the development of the microchip for computers revolutionized how we communicate and how we work throughout the world. Radio, telephones, and television changed how we communicated with each other and stayed abreast of what was going on in the world. The creation of the automobile, the assembly line, and airplanes transformed how we live, work, and travel. All of this and much more is due to technology. Historically, technology has presented human beings with objects that improved the quality of life, were time-saving, or prompted a broader view of possibilities. In almost all situations, technology has expanded our horizon.

Technological advances have supported health care trends and have taken us from a crude variety of methods to control or ease illness, injury, and disease to our current status. As the use of technology became more common in health care, an increasingly diverse selection of items and devices were developed, introduced, and then utilized to enhance health care practices. The use of some of these technological devices and advances are discussed in this chapter. Specific to occupational therapy is the use of assistive technology.

ASSISTIVE TECHNOLOGY

Assistive technology is defined as "any item, piece of equipment, or product system, whether acquired commercially off the shelf, modified, or customized, that is used to increase, maintain, or improve the functional capabilities of [individuals or] children with disabilities" (Woods, 2014).

Assistive technology can include the use of items to enhance living or remain in the home environment; the use of items to enhance student learning and doing at any age; items used to enable engagement within the parameters of any physical, developmental, sensory, or psychosocial challenge or limitation; items or equipment used to enable or enhance computer or cell phone use; items used to enhance driving ability; items used to facilitate rehabilitation goals (e.g., splints); and tool or item modification to facilitate a greater level of productivity, independence, or task engagement. Many occupational therapists use assistive technology to ease or hasten client engagement or reengagement in typical daily tasks. By being able to complete life tasks, people gain or regain the ability to assume their occupational roles.

Assistive technology can be further broken down into *low technology* and *high technology* categories.

Low Technology

A low-technology device for a child in the classroom can be something as simple as a pencil grip to ensure correct finger placement on a writing implement, or, in the case of an adult with arthritis, a low-technology item could be used to enlarge kitchen utensil handles or to pad tool handles for a construction worker with a weaker grip. Enlarging or padding on any item can increase the grip force, enlarge the gripping surface, and decrease discomfort or excessive stress on joints. Another simple example of low technology would be to color code the touch area for a microwave, round the edges of kitchen counters, or elevate the placement of a dishwasher. These things can be done at a relatively low cost and increase access to kitchen items. Low-technology items tend to be simpler in nature and less expensive (Woods, 2016) than items that include high-technology features.

High Technology

High-technology devices are generally more expensive and have some need for training and securing client skill or proficiency to use them correctly (Woods, 2016). For a child in grade school who has challenges in speaking or communicating with others, the use of an augmentative communication device would be a high-technology item. For an adult with physical challenges, a custom-fit wheelchair seating system used to improve sitting posture/position and environmental accessibility, along with the prevention of skin breakdown, would be considered a high-technology item. For older adults with compromised vision, the use of a screen reading text-to-speech or speech-to-text computer program is considered a high-technology item. For any smart phone user, text messages can be typed or dictated. For any individual with mobility and safety challenges, a tub enclosure with door access would assist in bathing, whereas the use of a stair lift would decrease the need to ascend and descend a stairway and ensure both client comfort and safety.

To summarize, technology is a component of independence for many clients. The therapist must know an item's availability, cost, and overall use to present, explain, demonstrate, observe, and review use with their client.

TECHNOLOGY USE IN OCCUPATIONAL THERAPY

The basic sequence of using any assistive technology is as follows:

1. Identify client need(s).
2. Identify available assistive technology options and vendors.
3. Identify the cost of the assistive technology item.
4. Determine whether the item will be reimbursable or covered through the client's health insurance, especially in the case of expensive items.
5. Assess whether the client is agreeable to using the item. (In the case of children or with clients who cannot make these kinds of decisions independently, assess whether the caregiver agrees to the purchase of the item.)
6. Once the item is secured, the therapist must review the item to ensure that he or she knows how to use and implement it to train or educate the client.
7. Present the item to the client with an explanation of what it is and how it is used.
8. If possible, demonstrate how the assistive technology item can be used.
9. Let the client use the item in your presence.
10. The occupational therapist trains and educates the client (and caregivers) in the correct and safe use of the item.
11. The client uses the item frequently and habitually within his or her daily life. Use of the item is safe and correct. This is frequently referred to as a *checkout*.
12. Once the item is automatically included in the client's daily routine, it can be considered a successful use of an assistive technology item.

The following three case studies represent the use of different types of assistive technologies. The first case study details the use of writing implements to enhance a child's grasp and prehension of a writing instrument. The use of these devices will enhance age-appropriate educational skills. The second case study includes the use of feeding devices designed to enable an adolescent to feed herself will less assistance. The third case study will include the use of higher technology items designed to enable a frail, cognitively challenged woman to reside and remain at home safely.

CASE STUDIES

Sam, a 6-Year-Old Boy

Sam's teacher and parents are concerned with his inability to print and write his name. The use of a pencil, pen, or marker are frustrating for him because of his inability to appropriately grip the writing device. Sam's peers laugh at the way he holds his pencil or pen. His ability to print his name is illegible and requires a good amount of energy and focus with poor results. Because of this, Sam is beginning to refuse to complete any assignment that requires writing or copying.

The occupational therapist is asked to perform a screen or to simply observe how Sam approaches a writing task. The occupational therapist observes that Sam is using his thumb, ring finger, and small finger as opposed to using the conventional thumb, index, and middle finger pattern.

The occupational therapist assesses Sam's functional range of motion in both hands, evaluates his grip strength and pinch strength, and has him use his thumb and index and middle fingers to pick marbles and paper clips out of TheraPutty (Fabrication Enterprises). He is able to use his hands functionally through this testing and activity. Based on these tasks, Sam also is using his left hand in a dominant manner. The occupational therapist then has him select colored markers to complete a simple coloring activity. When attempting to place the marker in his left hand, he begins to revert to the thumb, ring, and index pattern of prehension. The occupational therapist also notes that when holding the marker with his thumb, ring, and small fingers, he uses a "hook" wrist pattern. This wrist pattern is frequently seen in people who are left-hand dominant for writing or printing; this position also accounts for the heel of the hand getting soiled with the marker color or pencil carbon. The occupational therapist then provides colored pencils and another coloring task, along with a pencil grip. A pencil grip encourages correct finger placement using the thumb, index, and middle fingers. For left-handed individuals, the use of a left pencil grip also encourages a flatter wrist pattern and frequently will minimize or eliminate "hooking" of the wrist when printing, writing, or coloring. Although Sam reports that "this feels funny when I hold it," he agrees to use it when printing or writing and when coloring. The occupational therapist speaks with the teacher's aide, shows the aide the pencil grip and lets Sam demonstrate his use of the pencil grip. The occupational therapist asks the aide to have Sam use this grip in classroom activities and schedules a review of Sam's use of it in 2 weeks. This child's dysgraphia (handwriting difficulty without a neurological or intellectual disability) and poor pencil/pen grasp (or prehension) account for what is considered to be one of the most frequent reasons for occupational therapy referrals in the schools (Schwellnus, H., et al., 2012). As an initial intervention and use of low tech assistive technology, the pencil grip is frequently used as a tool to assist the individual in correct finger placement and to improve their sense of what the correct finger placement on a writing implement really is and what it feels like.

The occupational therapist returns for a review of Sam's left grip use and is pleased to discover that he is using it consistently to print, color, and write. The aide reports that he lost the original grip and that his parents purchased a package of left grips and brought them to school. He has used them consistently since that time. The aide also reports that Sam seems to have generalized this finger and thumb position when he uses thicker colored markers and when printing on the mark-and-wipe board in the classroom. The aide also states that Sam's parents purchased another package of grips for his use at home.

Sam's break-in period and generalization of the correct finger and thumb placement represent a successful outcome for the use of low-technology assistive technology. The use of a simple pencil grip has also allowed him to complete classroom and leisure tasks without any social or peer distress.

1. Why would the use of a pencil grip help Sam in both correct finger use and wrist positioning?
2. Why has Sam generalized his hand position for tasks other than printing and writing?
3. For Sam's age and stage, why is the use of the pencil grip decreasing the social and peer distress he was previously experiencing?

Hannah, a 15-Year-Old Girl With Cerebral Palsy

Hannah is a bright, friendly young woman who attends middle school locally. She experiences muscle tone fluctuations and difficulty feeding herself lunch and snacks in school. Her performance deteriorates at school due to having lunch with "the other normal students. I feel like a geek."

The occupational therapist is requested to observe her feeding skills in the school cafeteria to determine whether she is experiencing swallowing or chewing problems or if the problems relate to utensil use and positioning at the cafeteria table. The occupational therapist determines that Hannah's problems are the result of poor lunch table placement, the placement and type of food on her plate, her use of conventional feeding utensils (knife, fork, spoon) with an inconsistent grasp, and pronation-supination issues. Hannah also has difficulty raising feeding utensils to her mouth without losing or spilling the food content. As her occupational therapist, you assess her bilateral upper extremity active range of motion, assess her grip strength using a dynamometer, determine prehension and pinch strength using a pinch meter, and assess her joint flexibility through opposition and flexion-extension active range of motion testing. You also assess her ability to raise and lower the feeding utensil using foods with different consistencies, such as soup, pudding, applesauce, and salad, and with typical finger foods such as cheese crackers and nacho chips. Your occupational therapy evaluation takes place outside of the cafeteria in a quiet area of the classroom. Hannah states, "I don't feel so comfortable here. The kids look at me and laugh because I can't feed myself. That makes me feel so bad."

In your evaluation, you note that Hannah can raise a spoon, spork, or fork to her mouth with pudding, salad, and finer foods and achieves an almost perfect deposit of the food to her mouth. Her performance is compromised with liquid-type foods such as soup or applesauce. To use low-technology assistive technology items, you begin by enlarging the handle of a spoon using a foam grip enlarger (similar to small pipe insulation). The introduction of the enlarger seems to help Hannah attain a better grip on the utensil. When you try the grip enlarger with soup, the results are not satisfactory, and the soup dribbles onto the tabletop and over her chin, which embarrasses her. You then attempt to use a rocker spoon with an enlarged handle, and you make sure that her arms are supported by the tabletop. This results in less spilling of the liquid, but Hannah states, "I know this is better, but it's still messy." When using pudding, salad, and applesauce, her feeding performance is greatly improved by using the rocker spoon with the enlarged handle, however. When her arms are supported on the tabletop, she can independently feed herself finger foods. She reports, "I forget to place my arms on the table. When I don't, I run into trouble."

You determine the following:
- Hannah should be seated at the edge of the cafeteria table because there will be less distraction and potential noise.
- Hannah should have her arms supported on the tabletop.
- Hannah should practice using the swivel spoon with the enlarged handle both at school and at home.

You inform the teacher's aide, the cafeteria faculty member, and Hannah's teacher of the results of your evaluation.

Approximately 1 month later, you return to observe Hannah having lunch in the cafeteria at her school. She is seated at the end of the table, and is more appropriately seated in her chair with her arms supported. She is using the swivel spoon with the enlarged handle to feed herself cottage cheese with pineapple and a gelatin dessert, and she is using a conventional fork to eat a tuna salad. No problems are observed. The teacher's aide calls you aside and tells you that the "huge difference" at lunch is her table placement, her ability to automatically ensure that her arms are supported, the use of the spoon, and not getting soup or thin liquids to eat. The aide also reports that her parents have been pleased at her progress in feeding herself at home.

1. Why is positioning important for any feeding task?
2. What effect does arm support at the tabletop have for Hannah?
3. Why is it important to consider where she is seated at the cafeteria table?
4. Why would the introduction of a swivel spoon with an enlarged handle assist her?
5. Why would soup not be the best food item?

Marian, a 65-Year-Old Woman

Marian's grown children are concerned with her ability to remain in her beloved home due to her forgetfulness and their safety concerns. She recently forgot to turn off a stovetop burner and almost set her home on fire. Luckily, her neighbors saw smoke and rushed over to find a pot with burned food on fire on her stovetop. The neighbors put out the fire, and one of them contacted her children.

As an occupational therapist, you are called in by a home-care agency to perform a *home safety assessment* (HSA). An HSA is an in-home assessment in which the occupational therapist observes and assesses the living environment, methods of entrance and egress, steps, flooring, lighting, electrical issues such as cords, the height and width of items, carpets, bathrooms, storage, temperature, garage space, the presence of pets, and so on. The therapist then interfaces items with the client's current diagnosis, issues, and status. Please review the HSA at the end of this chapter (Box 8-1). Although this is a rather generic form of the assessment, it is thorough and can be made more specific depending on the situation.

Upon observing the home where Marian resides, you note that she must ascend or descend 10 steps to get from the outside to inside, and no railing is present. There is an attached garage, but it is used primarily for storage, and there is not enough space for a vehicle to park in its current state. If the garage were cleaned out, however, she would have only two steps to ascend or descend because the garage is connected to the interior kitchen. The kitchen has an older gas range with four burners, and the burners are turned on or off with dials located at the back of the stovetop. Although there is a cooking timer on the back of the stove, Marion reports that it does not work. A small microwave oven sits on her countertop. There is a porcelain sink across from the stove. The refrigerator sits on the back kitchen wall and is placed far away from the stove and sink. No dishwasher is present. You note that the appliances are older. The kitchen floor is ceramic tile and slippery. Marian reports that she was washing dishes earlier and forgot to mop up the floor. The handles on the cabinets are small and tend to stick rather than opening smoothly. You note that the small amount of counter space for food preparation is full of papers and grocery items that should be refrigerated but are not, and there is an open bag of dog food. Dog food and water bowls are sitting on the floor close to the oven door. Marian reports that the dog is outside in the fenced-in backyard. As you enter the dining room, you notice that there are electrical cords on the floor with throw rugs laying over them. The dining room also appears to be used as a storage area for papers, as papers and mail are randomly placed in piles throughout the space. The living room has a great deal of furniture and decorative items, again with many electrical cords on the floor covered by rugs. As you enter the living room, Marian stumbles over one of the electrical cords. There are 13 steps with a partial railing that lead you to the upstairs, where the only bathroom is located, plus three small bedrooms. Two of the bedrooms are full of clothing and other items. The bedroom that Marian uses is small and full of boxes and clothes. She has a "path" to her bed. Otherwise, there is no free floor space. The bathroom does not have a shower, only a tub, and she states, "I can only sponge bathe. I'm afraid to get in to the tub. I'm sure I would fall or not be able to either get in or out of the tub." The bathroom has a ceramic floor and three large rugs overlapping each other, and the tub is used for storage. The house also has a full basement, but Marian will not let you look in the basement "because it's full of junk."

1. From the information provided in the case study, identify the safety hazards that are present within Marian's home.
2. Based on this case study and the HSA findings, what would you determine the most important home safety issue to be?

3. What assistive technology items might increase the safety in the kitchen? In the dining and living rooms? In the bedroom where Marian sleeps? In the bathroom?

4. When considering safety, how could Marian get in and out of her home more safely, rather than reverting to the front entrance and the steps she must ascend (see Box 8-1)?

The HSA can be used to determine how the client functions within the home and can also be used to determine the need for assistive technology items within the home and respective rooms.

Frequent assistive technology items used within the home can include durable medical equipment (e.g., hospital bed, portable toilet, grab bars in the tub or around the toilet), the use of timers for the cooktop or oven (regular print size, large print size, or talking timers), water temperature thermometers, nonskid tub mats, anti-fatigue mats, angled pillows or height- and angle-adjustable beds, auto-close drawers, collapsible or folding walkers, talking clocks, universal remote controls, color-coded remote controllers for appliances or electrical items, enlarged grip kitchen items (e.g., hand mixers, knives), and many other things. Some assistive technology items bridge the gap between durable medical equipment and assistive technology. Regardless, if an item can be habitually used to increase safety and permit the client to perform daily occupations, the use is both meaningful and purposeful.

SUMMARY

Although the term *technology* can mean many things, for the purpose of occupational therapy, both low-technology and high-technology items are used as mainstream objects or things for the purpose of improving or increasing a client's engagement in occupations. The technology used varies from client to client. If a client is unable to perform an occupation or assume an occupational role, the therapist uses technology for learning and doing purposes. The use of technology also varies depending on the practice setting, the client's abilities or limitations, and frequently the availability or cost of the item. The therapist should consider these things to ensure the right fit with the client's age and stage of life, among other factors.

Box 8-1

HOME SAFETY ASSESSMENT

HOME SAFETY ASSESSMENT FORM

Name: _____   Date: _____

Address: _____

_____

Telephone Number: _____

Referred by: _____

Contact information of referral source: _____

Reason for HSA: _____

OUTSIDE

    a.   Method of entering home:

    b.   Steps with railing present?

    c.   Number of steps:

    d.   Are outside safety lights present?

    e.   Is a home security system present?

    f.   Are neighbors nearby?

INSIDE

Kitchen

    a.   Flooring present:

    b.   Types of appliances:

    c.   Placements of on/off dials or knobs or finger pads for appliances?

    d.   Can client demonstrate use of appliances?

    e.   Adequate counter space for food preparation?

    f.   Adequate storage for food items, dishes, utensils, countertop appliances?

    g.   Appliance and cabinet doors and drawers can be opened easily?

    h.   Adequate room for cooking and the cooking triangle is present (good interface between the sink, stove, refrigerator)?

    i.   Is adequate lighting present?

    j.   Does the stove have a vent fan?

(continued)

Box 8-1 (CONTINUED)

HOME SAFETY ASSESSMENT

Living and Dining Room or Area

a. Flooring present:

b. Furniture placement permits mobility throughout room?

c. As appropriate, is storage present?

d. Are throw rugs or electrical cords obvious? Does this deter safe mobility?

e. Can client independently and safely sit down and get up from furniture?

f. Is adequate lighting present?

Bedroom

a. Flooring present:

b. Does client sleep in designated bedroom? If not, where does the client sleep?

c. Adequate space to be mobile within bedroom?

d. Can client lie down and get up from bed independently?

e. Adequate storage present for clothes, shoes, other personal items?

f. Are throw rugs or electrical cords present?

g. Is there adequate lighting?

Bathroom

a. Flooring present:

b. Can client sit down and get up from toilet independently and safely?

c. Is a tub, shower, or tub and shower combination present?

d. Are grab bars present?

e. Is a moisture-venting fan present?

f. Is there adequate lighting?

Additional Home Spaces

Attic? Basement? Patio? Sunroom? Home office? Are there any safety issues in these spaces? Are/were you permitted to see these spaces? _____

_____

_____

Recommendations for HSA: _____

_____

_____

_____

_____

Signature: _____

QUESTIONS TO CONSIDER
FOR STUDENT LEARNING AND REASONING

These questions may help you learn and better visualize assistive technology items that are accessible and available in your community.

1. Are there any helpful or assistive devices you personally use regularly? Consider things such as glare-reducing screens on your computer or laptop, changing font sizes when you type assignments. When bathing or showering, do you use a washcloth and bar soap or a bathing sponge or net puff? Do you use bar soap or a gel? When brushing your teeth, do you use a manual or electric toothbrush? Is your clothing pull-on (e.g., yoga pants) or are zippers, buttons, or snaps used? Many of these daily-use items can be considered "assistive" because they make your life easier and allow you to perform daily tasks quicker and more efficiently.

2. Visit a local big box store or household goods store. Identify five "assistive" items you see, the reason for using these items, and their cost. Consider brands such as OXO kitchen items and the variety of kitchen devices with padded grips. Also look for bathing products, pain- or fatigue-reducing items, and easy-to-clean kitchen or bath products.

3. If possible, visit a local therapy clinic and watch the fabrication of a hand splint. Why is the splint being used for the client? What type of material is being used for the splint? Why is the splint being fabricated rather than commercially purchased?

REFERENCES

Oxford Dictionaries. (2018). Definition of technology. Retrieved from: http://www.Oxforddictionaries.com/definition/technology

Schwellnus, H., Carnahan, H., Kushki, A., Polatajko, H., Missiuna, C., & Chau, T. (2012). Effect of pencil grasp on the speed and legibility of handwriting in children. *American Journal of Occupational Therapy*, 66,6.

Woods, R. (2014). *Definition of assistive technology*. Retrieved from: http://www.gpat.org/Georgia-Project-for-Assistive-Technology/Pages/Assistive-Technology-Definition.aspx

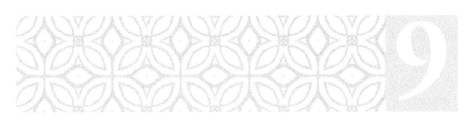

Future Initiatives
Programming for
the 21st Century

KEY WORDS

- *Centennial Vision*
- Demographics
- Emerging practice
- Epidemiology
- Evidence-based practice (EBP)

Hattjar, B.
Fundamentals of Occupational Therapy:
An Introduction to the Profession (pp. 127-143).

The title of this chapter, "Future Initiatives," is reflective of the dynamic and pro-active flow of the occupational therapy profession. The world is changing rapidly, and the profession of occupational therapy is following suit.

When considering the future of the profession, one must determine *demographics*, disease prevalence or *epidemiology, evidence-based practice* (EBP) or practice components, and the domain of the occupational therapy profession as a whole. Our professional domain is best viewed by looking at the breadth and scope of our *Occupational Therapy Practice Framework* (OTPF) (American Occupational Therapy Association [AOTA], 2014).

Demographics is defined as "relating to the study of changes that occur in large groups of people over a period of time, especially with regard to [population] density and capacity for expansion or decline" (Merriam-Webster Dictionary, 2018). The demographics of the United States indicate that people are living longer, health care promotes a more active and engaged "older age" for many people, the baby boomer generation has a distinctly different perspective of what "growing older" means than previous generations held, and although many older people choose to remain in their familiar home and town, others choose to move to different climates or closer to family or friends as they age and retire.

Epidemiology is the science that studies the patterns, causes, and effects of health and disease conditions in defined populations. Epidemiologists are public health professionals who investigate patterns and causes of disease and injury in humans (CDEC.org, 2018). They seek to reduce the risk and incidence of negative health outcomes through research, community education, and health policy (World Health Organization, 2015). Public health initiatives commonly include vaccinations, preventative resources designed to enhance life and reduce or eliminate the causes of illness, and the promotion of a more healthy and subsequently active lifestyle regardless of age.

EBP means applying the best available research (evidence) when making decisions about health care (Haughman, 2018). Health care professionals who perform EBP use research evidence along with clinical expertise and patient preference to guide services. In this situation, the practitioner is not only using EBP, but also a client-centered and holistic approach.

Professional domain of occupational therapy is best understood by reviewing the OTPF (AOTA, 2014). The OTPF provides practitioners with an overview of professional boundaries or parameters and the profession's depth and breadth. The OTPF also provides practitioners with common and frequently used vocabulary and terminology within the profession, commonly referred to as *professional jargon* (dictionary.com, 2005). It is prudent to remember that our clients and their caregivers many not understand our terminology, so it is always best to speak in terms that are well understood by the general population to avoid questions or misunderstandings.

These components represent areas that any program developer in any professional domain must consider. In the case for occupational therapy, demographics, epidemiology, and professional domain are crucial to consider and incorporate into initial programming, program development, and ongoing or established programs (due to the need to regularly evaluate program effectiveness).

THE PROCESS

Once these terms are understood and the scope of interest—the future—is determined, how can anyone determine where things are going for the profession of occupational therapy? To secure information, asking the right questions of the right people seems to be a plausible action to take. Therefore, 10 current occupational therapy practitioners and 42 occupational therapy graduate students were polled to determine what their personal experience comprises in the field. The graduate students completed their two professional-level fieldwork experiences within the previous year as of this writing. The practitioners had a total of at least 5 years and as much as 30 years of experience within the profession. Of the practitioners, three were occupational therapy assistants (OTAs) and seven were registered occupational therapists (OTRs). Data on this aspect of our professional future were captured from Pennsylvania, Ohio, Florida, Texas, Nevada, and New York through a convenience sample.

Those interviewed were asked the following questions (developed by the author):

1. Name the type of facility in which you work or in which you completed your Fieldwork II placement.
2. Identify the major diagnosis groups served in the facility (maximum of three).
3. Identify the types of occupational therapy assessments, evaluations, and screens conducted at this facility.
4. Identify the major types of occupational therapy interventions conducted at this facility.
5. State the average client length of stay or number of treatments that are conducted for a particular type of client or diagnosis at the facility.
6. Do you consider the interventions conducted at the facility to be "traditional" or "nontraditional, innovative, or emerging" types of services?
7. If you consider services to be traditional, please state why.
8. If you consider services to be nontraditional, please state why.
9. What areas do you feel are or will be emerging within the profession of occupational therapy?

The responses secured from the practitioners and graduate students were categorized according to traditional and nontraditional responses for interventions. Traditional interventions tended to occur, for this sample, in nursing homes, rehabilitation facilities, or hospitals. Nontraditional interventions tended to occur more frequently in outpatient or community-based facilities. Outpatient and community-based facilities were already viewed, according to the respondents, as facilities that conducted less traditional interventions, such as driver rehabilitation, work or industrial rehabilitation programs, low-vision programming, or health and wellness programming for older adults, children, and adolescents outside of a traditional hospital or nursing home type of setting, to name just a few. One community-based registered OTR respondent reported conducting living skills and communication programming, along with prevocational programming, for adults with a primary mental health diagnosis.

The polled group composition was as follows: 7 registered OTRs; 3 OTAs; and 42 graduate occupational therapy students (note that the professional practitioners saw clients related to their particular work setting, and the graduate students saw clients common to their Fieldwork II site placements).

Answers to Questions

Question 1: Name the type of facility in which you work or in which you completed your Fieldwork II placement.

- Psychosocial occupational therapy: 1 OTR; 2 students
- Rehabilitation facility: 3 OTRs and 1 OTA; 11 students
- Home care: 1 OTR and 1 OTA; four students
- Acute care: 1 OTR and 1 OTA; 11 students
- Nursing home or skilled nursing unit: 1 OTR; 14 students

Question 2: Identify the major diagnosis groups served in the facility (maximum of three).

One OTR working in the psychosocial realm of practice identified major diagnosis groups as follows: (a) depression, (b) post-traumatic stress disorder, and (c) anxiety disorders. The remaining six OTRs who work in traditional acute or skilled hospital units or rehabilitation facilities identified major diagnosis groups as: (a) cerebrovascular accidents (CVAs), (b) orthopedic problems (hip/knee replacements or hip fractures), and (c) traumatic brain injuries (TBIs).

The three OTA respondents identified (a) CVAs, (b) orthopedic issues (hip/knee replacement of hip fractures), and (c) general deconditioning issues.

Of the 42 graduate students polled, 25 reported the number one diagnosis seen during their Fieldwork II experience was CVA; 10 reported orthopedic issues; five reported autism spectrum disorders; and two reported TBIs.

The second most frequently seen diagnosis group for the graduate students included neurological issues (Parkinson's disease, multiple sclerosis), seen by eight students; arthritis or status post-upper extremity surgery rehabilitation, cited by 15 students; low-vision diagnoses, seen by five students; intellectual disabilities, seen by five students; and nine students saw clients with "balance," "safety," or "cognitive" problems. These comments were not specified for a particular diagnosis group.

The third most common diagnosis for the 42 graduate students included low back injuries seen by five students, feeding and swallowing problems seen by four students, general deconditioning issues seen by three students, vision problems seen by nine students dementia (including vascular and Alzheimer's type) seen by eight students, pain seen by five students, learning disabilities seen by five students, and three students did not provide a response.

Question 3: Identify the types of occupational therapy assessments, evaluations, and screens conducted at this facility.

The responses to this question for assessments or evaluations were as follows:

- Facility-based evaluations developed for a particular population
- The Kohlman Evaluation of Living Skills or the Functional Independence Measure
- The Canadian Occupational Performance Measure

These evaluations were used for a variety of client diagnosis groups and across age-groups.

Screens that were mentioned frequently include the Mini-Mental State Examination for both physical disability and psychosocial or mental health issues and the Allen Cognitive Level Screen (ACLS) for TBIs, the mental health populations, and people with cognitive problems. The ACLS was used frequently to determine clients' abilitiesto live independently, to assess safety, and to determine the best ability to function in a less restrictive environment, such as the home. Additional screens or questionnaires used as reported by both practitioners and students included pain scales and interest checklists. Although these two items are more of a general nature, three students reported that it gave them a good place to initiate treatment and helped them to converse with the client.

Question 4: Identify the major types of occupational therapy interventions conducted at this facility.

On the basis of all respondents' answers, the largest grouping of interventions included activities of daily living (ADL; e.g., dressing, bathing, grooming, or toileting); therapeutic exercise within a functional and purposeful activity; transferring and bed mobility; range of motion exercise and exercise in general; and functional household activities such as cooking, laundry, and cleaning. Only three respondents identified therapeutic crafts and two respondents reported communication skill development such as assertiveness training.

Question 5: State the average client length of stay or number of treatments that are conducted for a particular type of client or diagnosis at the facility.

Client diagnosis seemed to be the major factor in determining the length of stay at a given facility. Most respondents indicated that "more serious" or "life-threatening" illnesses resulted in a length of stay of 14 to 21 days in specialized or intensive care units, whereas other respondents indicated "1 to 2 weeks, but usually less" for postsurgical and orthopedic issues. Mental health and pediatric respondents indicated "less than 1 week", but this was dependent on medication management issues or the severity of the diagnosis.

Question 6: Do you consider the interventions conducted at the facility to be "traditional" or "nontraditional, innovative, or emerging" types of services?

The majority of the respondents reported that their interventions were more tradi-tional in nature overall. Respondents who indicated that more innovative or emerg-ing interventions were practiced were those practitioners or students who worked or completed Fieldwork II placements in places other than traditional hospitals or rehabilitation facilities.

Question 7: If you consider services to be traditional, please state why.

For those respondents who replied that interventions were traditional, they reported that their client work promoted increased client capacity for returning home. One respondent stated, "I provide interventions that I learned in school, and these things are what my clients need in order to get back home. Once they get home, they can personalize what they need in either home care or in outpatient. I just get them doing what they need to be able to do to get home."

Question 8: If you consider services to be nontraditional, please state why.

All respondents indicated that their "nontraditional or emerging services" were framed in their practice location more than by interventions being novel in nature. The respondents indicated that community-based services "seemed to be where the profession is heading rather than being confined in a hospital or clinic location." Home-care practitioners indicated that they promoted the clients' living at home by providing more client-centered and client-identified services based on need or by client or caregiver requests. Other respondents reported that they provided driving assessments, work-related assessments, or pediatric and sensory evaluations, all of which were considered to be either "new" or less well-defined by the profession.

Question 9: What areas do you feel are or will be emerging within the profession of occupational therapy?

Of all 52 respondents, 30 reported something along the lines of anything dealing with the aging population, such as low vision, driving rehabilitation or driver safety associated with the aging process, dementia, cognitive decline, orthopedic problems, and the concept of "aging in place." Ten respondents identified expanding our ability to work with either younger and chronically ill clients or with older and more fit but chronically ill clients in both traditional and community-based settings (including physically disabled and mentally ill clients). Ten of the respondents stated that the profession needs to become more adept in using physical agent modalities to provide a more comprehensive "menu" of intervention selections. Two respondents identi-fied improving how and where we provide services to children and adolescents, with community-based services identified as being important for occupational therapy to transition into. Both of these respondents indicated that "afterschool programming for adolescents" and "working with children and their parents" were paramount in interest and need.

COMMON THEMES

- Throughout this poll, one theme that seemed to be persistent was the need for occupational therapy involvement in varying prevention-related situations. This falls well in line with the Patient Protection and Affordable Care Act (PPACA, 2010). The ACA emphasizes preventative care not only to improve overall health, but to promote wellness through early interventions and patient health management to reduce chronic and costly diseases (PPACA, 2010). With the Patient Prevention and Affordable Care Act, the placement of occupational therapy in the prevention arena is of paramount importance. Prevention initiatives cover many areas, including education, monitoring progress, increasing client or patient awareness, inoculations, safety adherence to performance, adaptive device use, and so on. Prevention is usually determined by the population demographics, epidemiology, and evidence related to the particular situation, illness, or disease.

- Another common theme was the movement of the profession into either community-based settings or less traditional practice areas such as driver rehabilitation; vision; mental health recovery initiatives; home-based or aging-in-place settings for older adults; occupational role-based interventions such as work, homemaking, child care, school, or leisure venues; and engagement in end-of-life care (hospice).

- The need for some degree of skill improvement or updating was also a common theme. Items such as physical agent modalities; splinting (including both static and dynamic splinting); the use of creative and appropriate pieces of adaptive equipment; and a review or return to more historically based interventions such as crafts, cooking, and home management are noted.

- The students and practitioners who were polled indicated that there is a need for occupational therapy to "return to its roots" and develop a well-researched composite of information concerning what, how, and why particular intervention methods are selected. It was also mentioned that "insurance companies need to be educated" because reimbursement for some therapy interventions is difficult or impossible to bill for in the clinical setting. In this situation, being able to provide evidence of the effectiveness of the use of occupational therapy can be invaluable.

- The respondents frequently remarked that it is important for practitioners to realize the connection between clients' physical body and mind (also referred to as *thinking processes*). This mind-body connection means, literally and figuratively, that if one element of this dyad is "ill" or nonoperational, the other tends to follow.

Another option to gain a nationwide and professional view of what is emerging within our profession is to review *emerging practice* in occupational therapy via the AOTA website (Yamkovenko, n.d.).

AOTA currently has a list of potential emerging practice areas within the profession. These areas include:

- Children and Youth
- Health and Wellness
- Mental Health
- Productive Aging
- Rehabilitation and Disability
- Work and Industry

Additionally, AOTA has included "emerging niches" within each of these areas:

- Children and Youth: A broader scope within the school setting, childhood obesity, transition for older youth, bullying, teen driving
- Health and Wellness: Obesity, prevention, chronic disease management
- Mental Health: Depression, sensory approaches, recovery and peer support models, mental health dealing with veterans and wounded warriors
- Productive Aging: Alzheimer's disease and dementia, low vision, aging in place and home modifications, community mobility/older drivers
- Rehabilitation and Disability: Autism in the adult population, hand transplants and bionics, telehealth, cancer care and oncology, technology, veterans and wounded warrior care
- Work and Industry: Aging workforce, use of technology in the work setting

DO THESE POLL RESPONSES ALIGN WITH THE DIRECTION OF OCCUPATIONAL THERAPY IN THE *CENTENNIAL VISION*?

The *Centennial Vision* was proposed in 2003 to be a roadmap for the future of the profession to commemorate the AOTA's 100th anniversary in 2017 (AOTA, 2006). In 2006, a retreat of all of AOTA's component bodies, including the American Occupational Therapy Foundation; the National Board for Certification in Occupational Therapy; students; and a cross-section of practitioners, educators, scientists, and staff, participated in a strategic visioning retreat. The purposes of this retreat were to articulate a shared vision of the occupational therapy profession (AOTA, 2006). Additionally, strategic directions that were designed to guide the association and its members were set, and the hope that this endeavor would deepen the resolve to shape the future of the profession was promoted. At that time, a proposed shared vision statement was developed: "We envision that occupational therapy is a powerful, widely recognized, science-driven, and evidence based profession with a globally connected and diverse workforce meeting society's occupational needs" (AOTA, 2006).

When one maps the *Centennial Vision*, AOTA's emerging practice areas and niches, and the information that was secured in the poll taken by the author and presented in this chapter, it is clear to see that these three information areas are closely aligned.

Results Based on Comparisons of the Poll, AOTA's Emerging Practice Areas and Niches, and the Centennial Vision

- People are living longer and want to remain as healthy and involved as possible.
- People who have chronic diseases are diagnosed earlier due to improvements in health care.
- Concerns such as obesity and bullying are addressed earlier and in a more assertive and upfront manner; more options are provided to address such issues.
- The profession must keep up with technological advances such as bionics, ergonomics, and medication interaction and use.
- The skill set for therapists must encompass traditional and nontraditional service provision.
- Now more than ever, therapists must be able to teach both client and caregivers the "how, what, when, and where" of providing therapeutic interventions in a variety of client-familiar settings (e.g., home, school, while traveling).
- If a client need or needs are not adequately addressed by the profession, the therapist must have the tools necessary to develop appropriate client programming to provide services that address those needs.
- The therapist must have adequate knowledge of the anatomy and physiology of a client, along with knowledge of mental health, developmental, behavioral, and cognitive issues to provide truly holistic care in a wide variety of settings with a variety of age-groups.
- Therapists must be able to easily and quickly access information about disease, evaluation, intervention, and treatment strategies.
- Although the profession is advancing in a variety of specific areas, a therapist must have strong, basic skills before specializing to avoid tunnel vision and compartmentalization of knowledge and skills.
- It is the therapist's responsibility to remain current with directions and changes in health care.

EXPECTED EMERGING PRACTICE AREAS

The environment for occupational therapy services in the future is expected to be "more community-based" as opposed to being set in more traditional settings such as hospitals, clinics, or schools; this trend is already in evidence. A community base promotes and addresses the needs of specific communities and groups and promotes the development of new and more programs designed to enhance health and well-being.

Programs located in the community may or may not have an occupational therapist on staff. In fact, in many cases, occupational therapy is not yet or has not even been considered as a component of specific community programming. It is therefore important that occupational therapists have at least a basic knowledge of how to develop a community program to increase the likelihood of the inclusion of occupational therapy into community settings.

Community Programs: Basic Development

There is a basic and sequential approach for the development of community-based programs. It is important to "do your homework" by following these basic steps to ensure that the program is appropriate, needed, and wanted by the community agency and that it is based on facts—not just a great idea thought up over coffee! Linda Fazio (2008) called this basic process *profiling* or the *service profile*. The basic components of the service profile, provided in more detail in the numbered program development steps that follow, include determining (a) the population (who needs the service or program?), (b) the condition that is to be addressed, and (c) in what context the service or program will be presented or conducted.

Program development follows these steps in a more or less specific structure as follows:

1. Identify the community stakeholders. Stakeholders (a business and public health jargon term) are the people working at the agency or facility who have a presence or a role in the community agency.

2. Develop ongoing communication with the agency or facility. This can be initiated by a telephone call (a cold call, another business or public health jargon term) defined as an unsolicited telephone call in an attempt to sell goods or services. With this type of call, you are seeking to find out whether there is an interest or some level of motivation to proceed further. The best scenario for this telephone contact would result in the scheduling of a face-to-face meeting at a facility. Try to find out as much as possible about potential interest in programming at this time.

3. Develop a needs assessment that includes a review of the types of clients served at the agency, client ages and diagnoses (if appropriate), the days and times of current programming, and a clear determination of how occupational therapy can interface with the needs of the program or facility. At this stage, it is also important to determine any potential funding or grant sources that may be required to conduct the potential program.

4. After meeting in person, complete a literature review. This can be relatively easy to accomplish on the AOTA website (http://www.aota.org) or by completing a search in professional journals by searching, for example, key terms such as *wellness program for older adults* through a gerontology, social work, nursing, or occupational therapy journal or database, like PubMed or Psychnet, to name

just a few additional resources. If you are in an academic setting, a trip to the university library can be very helpful. Periodical areas within a university library will most likely provide a multitude of "hard copy" references. My experience tells me the information that can be secured in this manner is both current and relative to the specific population.

Conducting a literature review may seem unnecessary, and you may think it is a waste of time. Actually, the literature review can provide you with information concerning similar or duplicate types of programs throughout the United States. The literature review can also help to direct or hone in on specific program components that you may want to include. More than anything, the literature review can provide substantiation for the further development of your program.

5. Maintain open communication with your community facility and with the stakeholders. Keep these people abreast of how you are progressing and ask questions about your direction and their thoughts on your developing program.

6. Consider program supplies and major purchases necessary to execute the program. Be cautious and thoughtful in what you are identifying as "something needed" for the program to proceed, and always consider whether the program content would be diminished if the item or supplies were not purchases. However, another way to think about purchased, be they small or large, is that you may be more likely to secure larger ticket items at the beginning (referred to as *the honeymoon period*) than further down the line in the actual program execution.

7. Consider program staffing. Does your program require a large number of people to execute it, or can the program be done, for example, by supervised volunteers, supervised students, or current staff at the facility? In programs that have been started in my local area, they are generally developed by senior occupational therapy students and manned by junior students, all of whom are supervised by an OTR and on-site program staff. Many successful programs start small and build year after year. This slow development and the time allotment for program evolution has resulted in a greater likelihood that an occupational therapist will be understood and wanted by the facility to conduct programming.

8. At the onset of your program, it is crucial to put forth your vision of what the program will include during its first "run." By providing a linked and occupational therapy-based constellation of about 8 to 10 weekly groups, the overall progression of your program can be experienced by clients and reviewed by program stakeholders. This is helpful to everyone involved, especially if you are not going to be conducting the program. In this case, your diligence in planning and structuring your program can be provided to those individuals who will be conducting your program and your activities. This will get all those involved on the same page.

9. Link your program to occupational therapy. Your program should be occupation-based, purposeful, and functional. It should meet needs identified by the community program and the program clients. If this can be linked with the

doing, learning, and meaning components of the profession, you will have an occupational therapy-based program.

10. Provide a method of program evaluation. This aspect of program development can be daunting. Think about program evaluation like this: What do you anticipate the positive benefits to the participants might be? What do you anticipate will *not* happen if people participate in your program (i.e., can it help prevent negative outcomes)? For example, in an afterschool program designed for "latchkey" or underprivileged children, youth, and adolescents, positive benefits might include a decrease in legal altercations, reduced involvement in gang-related activities, or a decrease in sexual acting out, for example. In the case of an educationally based supportive program for the same individuals, you might anticipate that grades would increase by one letter grade or, at least, grades would not decline. A crucially important part of program evaluation is to make evaluation goals observable, measurable, and objective. Additionally, it is imperative that evaluation goals be attainable within the specific time period when the program is being conducted. Program evaluation is completed at the end of a program. This can be accomplished by objective evidence, such as report card grades; through stakeholder or participant completion of simple questionnaires; or by interviewing involved participants, stakeholders, or participant caregivers face-to-face. Program evaluation also provides the program providers with the opportunity to inquire about content that worked or did not meet participant needs, the need for programming changes, or to determine whether the program is actually needed and beneficial to the participants and to the facility.

11. Your completed program must be presented to your community stakeholders. It is also helpful to provide your stakeholders with a hard copy and an electronic copy of the complete program.

SPECIFIC EMERGING PRACTICE AREAS

This chapter has thus far addressed the context of programming for the future, and that context is the community-based program areas. The concept of the community is broad, and so are the various types of programs in which occupational therapy can and probably will provide services.

If we consider the areas identified by the AOTA as "emerging," future and emerging practice areas represent a diverse and ever-changing scope of professional service program provision.

Children and Youth

A large number of practitioners work with children and youth in a variety of settings and with a variety of skill sets. AOTA identified one major area that is becoming more prevalent in occupational therapy: working with children and youth diagnosed on the autism spectrum (American Psychiatric Association, 2013). These young people may be seen in the school setting, at home, in outpatient therapy, or in a mental health setting, among many other settings including the community. The number of people diagnosed with "autism" or "autistic-like" symptoms continues to increase. Autism Speaks, a national organization that promotes a greater understanding of autism, identifies that 1 in every 66 births results in a child who is autistic (Autism Speaks, 2015). It is interesting to note that this number has changed in as little as 10 years. In 2005, the number of children diagnosed with autism was 1 in every 166 births (Autism Speaks, 2015).

Another area that is emerging under the cfhildren and youth category is caseload to workload. This includes a full constellation of school-based practice comprising promotion, prevention, and intervention. This education and service-driven area also includes identification of the practitioner workload and the identification of the need for additional therapists for service provision (AOTA, 2015).

Another area in this category is early intervention, usually considered to be the provision of service from birth to 3 years of age. This includes preschoolers, toddlers, and their families and caregivers. Early intervention, in this situation, deals with the activities of daily living of play, rest, and sleep, as well as toileting, nap and sleep time, socializing, and education (AOTA, 2015).

The area of mental health in this young population is gaining more attention as practitioners realize that both the body and mind must be treated. In this specific population, promotion, prevention, school issues, bullying, social issues, and learning issues are highlighted (AOTA, 2015).

An important aspect of children and youth development is play. This includes the selection of appropriate toys, learning through play activities, the building of appropriate play skills, and appropriate use of school-related recess time (AOTA, 2015).

School-based practice focuses on academic achievement and educational relevance of therapy. This focuses on the learning or educational aspect of school-based services that are provided by the occupational therapist. In general terms, this encompasses work in the classroom (printing and writing, focus and attention, vision, hearing, posture, reading, math skills and concepts, the use of technology, the use of classroom tools like scissors, a ruler, etc.). Along with this major component, involvement in recess and gym time is also identified and focused on for this age-group. One additional area of focus is involvement in lunch and cafeteria activities, including feeding, balance, decreasing distraction, and social engagement (AOTA, 2015).

The use of the sensory integration approach to treatment is identified as another emerging area by the AOTA, which has indicated that there is a need for research and evidence-based proof of effectiveness using this theoretical approach. Sensory integration should be considered a "part of the intervention plan" when appropriate and used as a comprehensive approach rather than in bits and pieces vis-à-vis isolated components of the theoretical base (AOTA, 2015). In this case, this means that sensory integration must be a comprehensive part of the therapeutic intervention, not just a convenient or "add-on," such as a sensory diet or picking and choosing particular techniques.

Utilizing the occupational therapist to assist the child or youth deal with developmental transitions (e.g., elementary to junior high school, high school to work) or helping individuals deal with illness, injury, or loss figure prominently in this emerging component area (AOTA, 2015).

The last component of children and youth services involves youth transportation. This includes use of public transportation, riding a bicycle, preparation for driving, safe pedestrian mobility, the use of a car seat for younger children, and the use of safety devices such as seatbelts. In this area, it is important to determine what level of coordination is required and to what extent emotional regulation must be recruited to be both safe and well. Accessibility issues are also a component of this area (AOTA, 2015).

Health and Wellness

As a population, the United States has become more aware of the effect of both health and wellness on the maturation process. We are more aware of the effects of food, exercise, rest, engagement, and illness processes than ever before. This may be due to the easy access to health and wellness-related information on television and the internet, along with the fact that people have become more astute and educated consumers in this area.

This emerging area, according to AOTA (2015), comprises the following areas: physical and emotional health; the growing aging population, which is experiencing increased longevity; increased population awareness of health care disparity, which means that not all people have the same access to health care services for a variety of reasons; increasing obesity in the U.S. population overall; the use of technology and telehealth programs to increase access to health care and the monitoring of the disease and health processes; and the imbalance of roles within this area (e.g., some people follow a strict healthy lifestyle or see their physician regularly, whereas others do not maintain a healthy lifestyle and do not regularly visit their physician, even for routine checkups).

Mental Health

Mental health problems are one of the leading causes of disability in the United States. This emerging area encompasses mental health across the life span and is one area in which occupational therapy must become more involved. If you remember reading about the historical roots of the profession (Chapter 1), mental health treatment was one of the first major interventions areas for the fledgling profession (see also Chapter 2). Over the 20th century, occupational therapy's involvement in mental health decreased, but it is hoped that this is reversing today. A major focus of mental health interventions at this time is the recovery aspect. Many mental health problems can be surmounted and "recovered from" and do not have to be a lingering concern, just like many physical illnesses can be resolved or cured. The focus of work in this emerging (or reemerging) area includes intervening with serious mental illness and mental health problems; dealing with mental health issues in children, youth, adolescents, adults, and older adults; and working and intervening with depression

(AOTA, 2015). Depression is considered to be one of the leading causes of disability in the future (AOTA, 2015).

Productive Aging

The 2010 Census resulted in the following demographic information and future projections: in 2010, the over–65 population was estimated to be 43.1 million people as the first of the baby boomer generation (those born between 1945 and 1962) reached 65 years of age; by 2050, the estimated over-65 population will almost double in number to 83.7 million people in the United States (Ortman, Velkoff, & Hogan, 2014). AOTA (2015) identified the following components in this area as being relevant to occupational therapy:

- The aging population and the aging processes
- Increased longevity of the population
- The changing work world (people are no longer retiring at age 65 years; according to the U.S. Census Bureau, in 2010, those born between 1943 and 1954 will retire at "full retirement age"—the age when Social Security payments will be determined to be a full, not reduced, payment—at age 66 years. Those born between 1955 and 1959 can retire with "full" reimbursement in increments of 2 months per birth year [e.g., those born in 1955 will retire at age 66 years, 2 months and so on] until those born in 1960 and beyond can retire at age 67 years [Anspach, 2015].)
- The effect of the baby boomer generation and its impact on aging gracefully and aging in place with a more active lifestyle
- The intent and desire of the aging population to maintain the quality of life that they have grown accustomed to throughout their life span (AOTA, 2015)

Rehabilitation and Disability

As medical advances continue in health care, the use of rehabilitation services continues to increase. The need to promote a meaningful life in the face of any disability is better understood by a larger percentage of the population, and most people recognize the need for rehabilitation after an illness, injury, or disabling condition surfaces. AOTA (2014) identifies this emerging area as comprising the following: increased evidence and EBP, driving, ADL, home management and homemaking tasks, caregiving and child care, quality of life, and life participation. The driving element refers not just to driving skills, but also to driving cessation, alternative means of transportation, and the retention of autonomy and independence when no longer driving. In an unpublished capstone dissertation (A. Brzuz, in person interview, April 11, 2015), a program designed to guide older or impaired drivers to "prepare for" not driving was introduced and, as this textbook goes to press, is being researched longitudinally to determine the effectiveness of a driving cessation preparation course conducted in 2014.

Work and Industry

The concept of "work" has been a reality for humankind since the beginning of our history. Early cave dwellers completed necessary hunting and gathering work and documented this in cave wall paintings. The pyramids provided both an enduring edifice and a documented tale of how their creation appeased the Egyptian gods and pharaohs. Work activities became the themes of many Renaissance paintings and continue to provide us with a picture of life during that time. As nations became more industrialized, including the United States, work became a central focus of society and culture. As the United States has become more technologically savvy, work has taken on a somewhat different identity in which humans operate machines rather than completing heavy or dangerous tasks by sheer force and body strength. People are working gainfully into their sixth decade. This presents issues with aging, sensory deficits associated with the aging process, and the need to retain a work identity and financial security. Work provides individuals with "economic rewards, meaning, and fulfillment" (AOTA, 2015). If work has and retains a positive effect on the worker, it can make life fulfilling. However, if work begins to take on a negative connotation, it can be detrimental to both the worker and the work environment. AOTA (2015) identifies work and industry components of the aging workforce and the need to develop compelling evidence for occupational therapy's involvement in this area.

SUMMARY

The constellation of emerging practice areas encompasses the same wide body of knowledge evidenced by the occupational therapy profession. It provides us with a testimony of our profession's adept skill at addressing both current and future needs and our ability to promote a holistic and purposeful complement of services to our current and future clients. If occupational therapy remains consistent in both being mindful of today while planning for the future, the profession's credibility in health care will be solidified, and the need for occupational therapy services will continue to grow in the future.

REFERENCES

Allen Cognitive Group. (2018). Welcome. Retrieved from: http://www.allencognitivecom

American Occupational Therapy Association. (2006). *AOTA's Centennial Vision.* Retrieved from https://www.aota.org/-/media/corporate/files/aboutaota/centennial/background/vision1.pdf

American Occupational Therapy Association. (2014). *Occupational therapy practice framework.* Retrieved from https://ajot.aota.org/article.aspx?articleid=1860439

American Occupational Therapy Association. (2015). *Wellness and productive aging: Fact sheet.* Retrieved from https://www.aota.org/Practice/Productive-Aging.aspx

American Occupational Therapy Association. (2015). *Emerging practice niches.* Retrieved from https://www.aota.org/Practice/Manage/Niche.aspx

American Psychiatric Association. (2013). *The diagnostic and statistical manual of mental disorders* (5th ed.). Washington, DC: Author.

Anspach, D. (2015). *Average retirement age in the United States.* Retrieved from http://moneyover55. about.com/od/preretirementplanning/g/Average-Retirement-Age-In-The-United-States.htm

Autism Speaks. (2015). *Autism facts.* Retrieved from https://www.autismspeaks.org/what-autism/ facts-about-autism

Centers for Disease Control and Prevention. (2018). Principles of Epidemiology in Public Health Practice, An Introduction to Applied Epidemiology and Biostatistics (3rd ed.). Retrieved from https://www.cdc.gov/ophss/csels/dsepd/ss1978/lesson1/section1.html

Dictionary.com. (2005). *Jargon.* Retrieved from http://www.dictionary.com/browse/jargon?s=t

Effective Health Care Program, Agency for Healthcare Research and Quality. (2015). Evidence-based practice definition and examples. Retrieved from http://effectivehealthcare.ahrq.gov/index.cfm/ glossary-of-terms

Fazio, L. (2008). *Developing occupation-centered programs for the community* (2nd ed.). Upper Saddle River, NJ: Pearson/Prentice Hall.

Haughman, J. (2018). *5 Reasons the Practice of Evidence-Based Medicine is a Hot Topic.* Retrieved from: http://www.healthcatalyst.com

Kohlman-Thompson, L. (2016). *Kohlman Evaluation of Living Skills (KELS),* 4th ed. Bethesda, MD: AOTA Press.

Law, M., Baptiste, S., Carswell, A., McCall, M., Polatojko. H., & Pollock, N. (2018). The Canadian occupational performance measure (COPM). Retrieved from: http://www.thecopm.ca

Merriam-Webster Dictionary. (2018). *Demographics.* Retrieved from http://www.merriam-webster. com/dictionary/demographic

Ortman, J. M., Velkoff, V. A., & Hogan, H. (2014). *An aging nation: The older population in the United States.* Washington, DC: U.S. Census Bureau. Retrieved from https://www.census.gov/ prod/2014pubs/p25-1140.pdf

PPACA. (2010). Patient Protection Affordable Care and Health Care and Education Reconciliation Act. 11th Congress 2nd Session. Retrieved from: www.healthcaregov/where-can-I-read-the-affordable-care-act/

Physio-pedia. (2018). Functional Independence Measure. Retrieved from: http://www.physio-pedia. com

Serwe, K., & Schultz, S. (2014). Fieldwork opportunities for enhancing occupational therapy's role in preventative care. *Education Special Interest Section Quarterly, 24,* 1–4.

University of Massachusetts. (2018). Mini-mental state examination (MMSE). Retrieved from the University of Massachusetts Lowell http://www.umi.edu/docs/Mini%20Mental%20State%20 Exam-tcm18-16931apdf

Wikipedia. (2015). *Epidemiology.* Retrieved from https://en.wikipedia.org/wiki/Epidemiology

World Health Organization. (2015). *Health topics: Epidemiology.* Retrieved from http://who.int/ topics/epidemiology/en

Yamkovenko, S. (n.d.). *The emerging niche: What's next in your practice area?* Retrieved from https:// www.aota.org/Practice/Manage/Niche.aspx

Index